Low-FODMAP Cookbook

1000 Days of Recipes to Alleviate IBS Symptoms. 4 Week Meal Plan Included.

Sophia Ciotti

SUMMARY

Chapter 1: Introduction

Step into a world of culinary exploration with a diet that can transform your health and lifestyle—the low-FODMAP diet. Whether you're Mike, a fitness enthusiast aiming to control his IBS symptoms, or Sarah, a proactive mother and career woman seeking to elevate her family's health and expand her dietary knowledge, this chapter is your first step.

Let's dive right into what FODMAP is and explore the fascinating science that underpins it. This exploration paves the way to understanding the significant connection between FODMAP and Irritable Bowel Syndrome (IBS). Next, we'll dive deeper into how FODMAP influences IBS and peruse the research affirming the effectiveness of the low-FODMAP diet in managing these symptoms. What comes out of this is a clear picture of the benefits a low-FODMAP diet can offer.

Now, imagine a diet that not only manages IBS but also provides health benefits that extend beyond it. Yes, it's the same low-FODMAP diet, and we'll uncover these benefits. As we move forward, we will walk you through how to utilize this cookbook to its fullest, from maneuvering the recipes to getting the hang of the meal plan. Thus, this chapter serves as a comprehensive guide, setting the stage for a transformative journey with the low-FODMAP diet.

Understanding FODMAP

What is the recipe for a healthy gut? It seems to be a question with no single answer, as scientists and nutritionists grapple with unraveling the complexities of our digestive system. However, a new contender has recently entered the ring of gut health contenders: FODMAP. An acronym for Fermentable Oligosaccharides, Disaccharides, Monosaccharides, and Polyols, FODMAPs are specific types of carbohydrates that some people struggle to digest properly. The result? Uncomfortable and sometimes debilitating symptoms for those with a sensitive gut or conditions like Irritable Bowel Syndrome (IBS). Let's take a closer look.

FODMAPs are present in an array of everyday foods, ranging from apples and pears to bread and pasta, onions and garlic to milk and yogurt. As a group, they are highly fermentable – meaning that when they reach the large intestine, the gut bacteria rapidly ferment them. For many individuals, this fermentation process can cause symptoms such as bloating, abdominal pain, constipation, diarrhea, or a combination of these.

When we digest our food, it travels from the stomach into the small intestine, where most of the digestion and absorption of nutrients takes place. If certain substances like FODMAPs aren't adequately digested and absorbed in the small intestine, they continue along their journey to the large intestine or colon. Here, they become a feast for the trillions of bacteria that call our gut their home. As these bacteria ferment the FODMAPs, they produce gas, resulting in bloating and discomfort.

Simultaneously, FODMAPs can also draw water into the intestine, contributing to feelings of distention, and potentially leading to diarrhea. On the flip side, in some people, these changes may slow down the transit time, leading to constipation. So, it's clear how these substances could create the perfect storm of digestive discomfort.

Consider this scenario: John, a 30-year-old financial analyst, has been suffering from digestive issues for a while. Every time he eats an apple as a mid-afternoon snack or has garlic in his dinner, he experiences bloating, abdominal pain, and uncomfortable changes in his bowel movements. However, when he replaces his apple with a banana and avoids garlic in his meals, his symptoms improve. This pattern is a typical example of how certain foods containing FODMAPs can lead to digestive discomfort in susceptible individuals.

Meanwhile, Sarah, a 35-year-old nutritionist and mother of two, might notice that her kids often complain of a stomach ache after eating ice cream or drinking milk – a sign of lactose, a disaccharide and a kind of FODMAP. Sarah herself might feel bloated and uncomfortable after having pasta for dinner – a meal high in wheat, an oligosaccharide, another type of FODMAP.

These scenarios are just a few examples of how FODMAPs might manifest themselves in everyday life. However, it's essential to remember that everyone's gut is different. What might cause discomfort for John might not affect another person, such as his gym buddy, the same way.

Understanding FODMAPs and how they interact with our gut is the first step towards a solution to the puzzle of digestive health for many people. It's the beginning of a journey towards taking control of your health and wellbeing. The goal is not to eliminate FODMAPs entirely from the diet – they have their health benefits, too – but to understand which ones might be causing you trouble and to manage them in a way that brings you the greatest comfort.

In this cookbook, we'll delve deeper into the world of FODMAPs, exploring how they could be affecting your gut health, and provide you with delicious, low-FODMAP recipes to help you on your journey towards a healthier, happier gut. So, whether you're like John, who's trying to manage his IBS symptoms, or like Sarah, who wants to improve her family's health through diet, understanding FODMAPs is the first step. The rest of the journey – full of delicious foods and a healthier lifestyle – awaits.

What is FODMAP?

Diving deeper into the world of FODMAPs, we need to decode what this acronym stands for: Fermentable Oligosaccharides, Disaccharides, Monosaccharides, and Polyols. Quite the mouthful, isn't it? However, don't let the science-y name scare you. Each part of this term has a specific meaning and understanding it can illuminate how these substances function and why they might cause discomfort for some people.

Let's break it down:

Fermentable refers to the process through which gut bacteria break down undigested carbohydrates to produce gases, including hydrogen, carbon dioxide, and in some people, methane. It's this fermentation process that can cause bloating and gas in susceptible individuals.

Oligosaccharides are complex carbohydrates, including fructans and galacto-oligosaccharides (GOS). They're found in various foods, including wheat, rye, onions, garlic, and legumes.

Disaccharides, specifically referring to lactose in the context of FODMAPs, are found in dairy products such as milk, cheese, and yogurt. Lactose intolerance is a well-known issue many people face, and it's due to the body's inability to break down lactose efficiently.

Monosaccharides refer primarily to fructose when we speak about FODMAPs. Fructose is a simple sugar found in many fruits, honey, and high-fructose corn syrup. Some people struggle to absorb fructose, which can lead to symptoms of abdominal discomfort.

Polyols are sugar alcohols and include substances like sorbitol and mannitol. They're found in some fruits and vegetables and are often used as artificial sweeteners.

Consider this, John, our financial analyst from the previous example, loves having apples as part of his lunch. However, he often finds himself feeling bloated and uncomfortable afterward. Apples, unbeknownst to John, are high in both fructose (a monosaccharide) and sorbitol (a polyol). These are two types of FODMAPs that his body might struggle to digest and absorb, leading to his unpleasant symptoms.

Meanwhile, Sarah, our nutritionist mom, enjoys a smoothie with her breakfast, usually made with a blend of fruits and a generous splash of yogurt. However, she often feels bloated afterward, causing her discomfort throughout her busy morning. The yogurt in her smoothie is rich in lactose (a disaccharide), which could be the culprit behind her digestive woes.

What makes FODMAPs particularly interesting is their diversity and ubiquity. They're not limited to 'unhealthy' foods or foods that you might typically associate with digestive discomfort. Instead, they're scattered across various food groups, encompassing fruits, vegetables, grains, legumes, and dairy products.

What makes these groups of carbohydrates even more fascinating is how they interact with our gut and our gut bacteria. They are fermentable, meaning that they're a favorite food of the bacteria in our gut. As the bacteria feast on these carbohydrates, they produce gas, which leads to the bloating and discomfort many individuals with IBS or a sensitive gut experience.

Learning about FODMAPs and their role in our diet and gut health isn't merely academic. It's a critical first step in understanding why certain foods may cause discomfort and how to manage that through dietary changes. For John, who is looking to control his IBS symptoms, understanding what FODMAPs are is a game-changer. It allows him to make informed dietary choices, managing his symptoms while still enjoying a rich and varied diet.

And for Sarah, who wants to improve her family's health and further her knowledge about diets, understanding FODMAPs provides her with a new tool. It offers a deeper insight into how food can affect our bodies and gives her the knowledge she needs to make healthful choices for herself and her family.

FODMAPs, although complex in their scientific nature, need not be intimidating. Understanding what they are and how they interact with our bodies can empower us to take control of our gut health and lead us on the path to dietary comfort and happiness. From oligosaccharides to polyols, each part of the FODMAP acronym is a piece of the puzzle of understanding our gut health, setting us on the journey of discovery and wellness.

The Science Behind FODMAP

Now that we understand what FODMAPs are, let's explore the science behind them and their impact on our digestive system. This understanding will provide a strong foundation to our journey into managing IBS and other digestive discomforts effectively.

Our digestive system is designed to break down the foods we eat into their smallest components for absorption. For instance, proteins break down into amino acids, fats into fatty acids, and carbohydrates into simple sugars. This process allows nutrients to be absorbed into our bloodstream and transported to cells throughout our body.

FODMAPs, however, present a unique challenge. They're a group of carbohydrates that are either not broken down or not absorbed well in the small intestine. As a result, they move along to the large intestine, where they become a food source for the bacteria that reside there. When these bacteria ferment FODMAPs, they produce gas, which causes the familiar bloating and discomfort associated with IBS and other digestive disorders.

Take John, for example, who is seeking to manage his IBS symptoms. After eating a large pasta meal with a garlic-infused sauce, he might experience abdominal discomfort, bloating, and other IBS symptoms. The pasta, made from wheat, contains fructans (a type of oligosaccharide), and the garlic is another high-FODMAP food. The fructans aren't well-absorbed in John's small intestine, leading to fermentation in the large intestine, causing gas and leading to his symptoms.

On the other hand, Sarah, keen on enhancing her family's health, might notice her children sometimes experience stomachaches after enjoying large fruit salads. Many fruits contain fructose (a monosaccharide) and some also contain sorbitol (a polyol), both of which can cause digestive discomfort when consumed in large amounts.

It's important to note that not everyone is sensitive to FODMAPs. Many people can consume high-FODMAP foods without experiencing any discomfort. However, for individuals with IBS or similar conditions, reducing the intake of FODMAPs can have a substantial impact on their symptoms and overall quality of life.

Understanding the science behind FODMAPs can aid in appreciating the rationale of a low-FODMAP diet. It empowers us to make informed decisions about our food choices, focusing on not only the nutritional value but also the potential effects on our gut health.

As we delve deeper into this fascinating world of FODMAPs, remember that knowledge is power. The more we understand our body and how it interacts with the food we eat, the better equipped we are to manage our health. Whether you're aiming to control your IBS symptoms like John or striving to make healthier dietary choices for your family like Sarah, understanding the science behind FODMAPs will be a cornerstone to your dietary success.

The Connection Between FODMAP and IBS

Irritable Bowel Syndrome, or IBS as it's commonly known, is a complex and often misunderstood condition that affects millions of people worldwide. For those living with IBS, the quest for dietary solutions can seem overwhelming. That's where the relationship between FODMAPs and IBS comes into play.

IBS is characterized by recurring symptoms like abdominal pain, bloating, and changes in bowel habits - diarrhea, constipation, or a combination of both. Although these symptoms can vary greatly from person to person, many people with IBS have one thing in common: a hypersensitive gut.

Imagine the gut as a pathway, starting at the mouth and ending at the anus. Along this pathway, our food gets broken down, absorbed, and eventually excreted. For people with IBS, their gut can be overly responsive to stimuli. Something as simple as eating a meal can trigger the gut to contract too forcefully or too weakly, leading to symptoms like pain, bloating, and altered bowel habits.

The gut's hypersensitivity is where FODMAPs come into the picture. FODMAPs are poorly absorbed in the small intestine and reach the large intestine, where they are fermented by gut bacteria. This fermentation process produces gas, leading to bloating and abdominal discomfort. Additionally, FODMAPs can draw water into the gut, leading to loose stools and diarrhea, particularly problematic for people with a hypersensitive gut, like those with IBS.

So, for someone like John, who enjoys dining out with friends, a meal at an Italian restaurant could result in a sleepless night filled with IBS symptoms. The wheat in the pasta, the onion and garlic in the sauce, and the apple in the dessert all contain high levels of FODMAPs. These compounds can trigger his gut to react, leading to a flare-up of IBS symptoms.

Similarly, Sarah's family might experience digestive discomfort after a family barbeque, where they enjoyed sweet sauces, beans, and coleslaw. All these foods are rich in FODMAPs and may provoke gut symptoms in individuals with IBS or FODMAP sensitivity.

Therefore, understanding the connection between FODMAPs and IBS is the first step towards regaining control over your health and your life. In the following chapters, we'll delve further into how to manage your or your family's diet to minimize IBS symptoms, focusing specifically on the role of FODMAPs. This knowledge is the key to unlocking a healthier, more comfortable life for people like John and Sarah and potentially for you and your loved ones.

How FODMAP Affects IBS

Living with IBS can feel like walking a tightrope. On the one hand, there's the desire to enjoy a varied and flavorful diet. On the other, there's the need to avoid the triggering of uncomfortable, and sometimes debilitating, IBS symptoms. Understanding how FODMAPs affect IBS can provide essential guidance for maintaining balance on this tightrope.

So, what exactly happens when FODMAPs interact with a gut prone to IBS?

Let's start by imagining the journey of FODMAPs through the digestive system. After being consumed, they travel through the stomach and into the small intestine, a crucial location for nutrient absorption. However, due to their particular structure, FODMAPs are poorly absorbed in the small intestine. Instead, they continue their journey largely intact into the large intestine, where our gut microbiota resides.

Once FODMAPs reach the large intestine, they act as fuel for the gut microbiota, undergoing a fermentation process. This fermentation leads to the production of gases, such as hydrogen, carbon dioxide, and in some cases, methane. In a normal gut, these gases can be comfortably managed. However, in an IBS-prone gut, the story is quite different.

Remember, an IBS-prone gut tends to be hypersensitive. The gas produced during fermentation can lead to the stretching of the intestinal walls, triggering discomfort, bloating, and pain. It's akin to a balloon slowly inflating, the pressure building up until it becomes unbearable.

But it's not just gas. FODMAPs, especially those that are osmotic, such as lactose and fructose, can draw water into the gut. This water influx can contribute to feelings of bloating and can lead to diarrhea, as the additional water speeds up transit in the gut.

So, when John enjoys his favorite pre-gym smoothie packed with high-FODMAP fruits, he might experience bloating and discomfort due to these combined effects. For Sarah, the issue might arise when she prepares a family meal rich in high-FODMAP ingredients. The resulting discomfort and bloating might leave her family feeling less than their best.

By understanding the specific ways that FODMAPs affect IBS, both John and Sarah can start to make more informed choices. The science behind FODMAPs is not about limiting enjoyment of food. Instead, it's about empowering individuals to understand how different foods can affect their bodies and make decisions accordingly.

In essence, knowledge of FODMAPs' impact on IBS is not about taking foods away; it's about providing the tools to add more symptom-free days to your life. This understanding could be the key that unlocks the door to a more comfortable and symptom-free life for those suffering from IBS.

Studies Supporting the Low-FODMAP Diet

It's always reassuring to know that when you make a dietary change, you're not going in blind. You want to know that there is a solid body of research to back up your decisions, something that our friend John, the fitness enthusiast with IBS, appreciates. John likes to research, he likes to understand the science before making any dietary changes that could affect his performance. He needs assurance that this isn't another fly-by-night fad. Similarly, Sarah, the health-conscious mother, wants to be sure she's making an informed choice when modifying her family's diet.

So, what does the science say about the low-FODMAP diet?

Numerous studies have been conducted over the years that provide concrete support for the use of a low-FODMAP diet in managing IBS symptoms. A significant example of this is a research study conducted by a team at Monash University in Australia. Their rigorous and meticulously designed study found that 74% of the participating IBS patients reported substantial improvement in their symptoms when following a low-FODMAP diet.

In another study published in the 'Gastroenterology & Hepatology' journal, a low-FODMAP diet was shown to effectively reduce symptoms in approximately 86% of patients with IBS, a percentage higher than any other dietary intervention.

Other studies have revealed similar promising results. A research study published in the 'American Journal of Gastroenterology' indicated that a low-FODMAP diet effectively reduced functional gastrointestinal symptoms in IBS patients. Patients in this study reported improvements in overall abdominal pain, bloating, and improved quality of life.

Beyond studies focused on IBS, research has also indicated that a low-FODMAP diet could be beneficial for individuals suffering from other functional gastrointestinal disorders. In fact, a study in the 'Journal of Gastroenterology and Hepatology' demonstrated that patients with inflammatory bowel disease (IBD), who also had IBS symptoms, experienced significant improvements in their symptoms after following a low-FODMAP diet.

These studies and others like them are crucial in the ongoing development and refinement of the low-FODMAP diet. They provide us with a substantial body of evidence that the low-FODMAP diet can, and does, help many individuals manage their IBS symptoms more effectively.

So, when John asks himself if the low-FODMAP diet is worth trying, he can find reassurance in these scientific studies. And when Sarah wonders if this diet could help her family, she too can find comfort in the accumulated evidence.

However, the studies are not just there to convince John, Sarah, or any potential followers of the low-FODMAP diet. They also guide healthcare professionals in their recommendations. When doctors, dietitians, and other healthcare providers recommend a low-FODMAP diet, it is not a shot in the dark; it's a recommendation supported by strong, scientific research.

Armed with this knowledge, you can approach a low-FODMAP diet with confidence, knowing it's not just another dietary trend, but a scientifically backed approach to managing IBS symptoms.

Benefits of a Low-FODMAP Diet

A diet is much more than just a way to control your weight; it's a lifestyle choice that affects every part of your life, from your physical health to your emotional well-being. Making the shift to a low-FODMAP diet is no different. It comes with numerous benefits, much beyond the obvious relief from IBS symptoms.

The low-FODMAP diet has been consistently associated with a significant reduction in symptoms of IBS, including abdominal pain, bloating, and altered bowel habits. These are the most immediate benefits that draw people like Mike to try this diet. The ability to exercise without the constant fear of triggering IBS symptoms can be a game-changer for Mike's fitness goals. It allows him to stay focused, build resilience, and maintain his active lifestyle, without IBS holding him back.

But it's not only about physical discomfort. Imagine the mental relief that comes from knowing you can eat a meal without worrying about how your body will react. For many IBS sufferers, a low-FODMAP diet can mean the difference between constant worry over every bite and a peaceful, enjoyable meal. For Sarah, knowing she's serving her family meals that won't trigger discomfort or pain brings her immense satisfaction.

Beyond IBS, emerging research suggests that a low-FODMAP diet might have benefits for other gastrointestinal disorders, like inflammatory bowel disease (IBD). While further research is necessary, early results are promising. If your health journey includes these conditions, a low-FODMAP diet may provide some additional benefits.

From a broader perspective, embarking on a low-FODMAP diet can also help individuals develop a more mindful approach to eating. It promotes awareness about how different foods affect the body and encourages a more in-depth understanding of food and nutrition. For someone like Sarah, who aims to broaden her knowledge about different diets, adopting a low-FODMAP lifestyle can be an enlightening experience.

Moreover, as one navigates the intricacies of a low-FODMAP diet, they also develop a healthier relationship with food. They learn to view food not just as a source of pleasure, but as nourishment, medicine, and a tool to manage their health.

Ultimately, the benefits of a low-FODMAP diet go beyond the confines of a dining table or a meal plan. It influences your lifestyle, your approach towards health, and your perception of food. It's about enhancing your quality of life, improving your physical health, and nurturing your emotional well-being.

Embarking on a low-FODMAP journey might seem daunting at first glance, but once you start experiencing the benefits, you realize it's not just about what you lose (the high FODMAPs), but more about what you gain - control over your health, freedom from discomfort, peace of mind, and a greater understanding of your body and its relationship with food.

Health Benefits: Beyond the Digestive Tract

A low-FODMAP diet is known for its immediate effects on gut health, reducing the symptoms of IBS and enhancing digestive comfort. But, just like a ripple effect, the benefits extend far beyond the digestive system.

Firstly, the low-FODMAP diet can play a significant role in weight management. Now, it's not a weight-loss diet, per se. It doesn't promise a drastic reduction in pounds. However, it does promote mindful eating and healthier food choices, which can help you maintain a balanced weight. Remember, a stable weight isn't just about looking good for the beach season; it's about heart health, joint health, and overall vitality. For someone like Mike, this aspect of weight management could tie in well with his fitness goals.

Secondly, a low-FODMAP diet can boost your immune system. An interesting fact is that the majority of our immune system is located in our gut. So, if your gut health improves, so does your immunity. Less inflammation in the gut means less overall stress on your body, freeing up your immune system to fight off actual threats, like viruses and bacteria. In this era, who wouldn't appreciate an extra layer of immune defense?

Next, the low-FODMAP diet can also be an ally in your mental health journey. The gut and the brain are connected via the gut-brain axis, and what affects one can influence the other. If your gut is in distress, it can send signals of discomfort to your brain, potentially leading to mood changes and heightened stress. On the other hand, a happy gut can contribute to better mental well-being. For someone like Sarah, this could mean better handling of work stress and more patience when dealing with her family.

Additionally, a low-FODMAP diet can also contribute to better sleep. Reduced nighttime discomfort can lead to better quality sleep, and good sleep is integral to overall health. From mental clarity to heart health, good sleep is a non-negotiable for optimal health.

Last but not least, a low-FODMAP diet promotes overall nutritional balance. Many low-FODMAP foods are nutritionally dense, packed with essential vitamins, minerals, and antioxidants. These nutrients are the building blocks of health, supporting everything from skin health to brain function.

So, when we talk about the health benefits of a low-FODMAP diet, we're not just talking about the gut. We're talking about your entire body, your mind, your daily performance, your mood, your sleep, your immunity, and so much more. Adopting a low-FODMAP diet, then, is not just about eliminating certain foods; it's about embracing a holistic way of living that has your overall health at its heart.

Lifestyle Benefits: The Silver Lining of a Low-FODMAP Diet

While the low-FODMAP diet has been primarily designed to alleviate digestive symptoms, the lifestyle benefits it bestows are profound and far-reaching. Our friends Mike and Sarah, each with their distinct goals, would find the versatility of these benefits quite compelling.

For Mike, with his focus on fitness and managing IBS, the low-FODMAP diet might come as a gift. By reducing digestive discomfort, he'd discover that his energy levels are more consistent, leading to more efficient workouts. No more feeling sluggish during his runs or half-hearted during his gym sessions. Instead, he could enjoy a newfound sense of vitality, allowing him to engage more dynamically in his routine physical activities.

Moreover, a clearer mind is a notable spin-off of a healthier gut. Without the constant nagging of an upset stomach, Mike could concentrate better on his professional commitments and personal growth. Imagine the freedom of not having to plan your life around restroom availability or cope with the nagging pain of a bloated belly. Mike would likely find his overall quality of life considerably improved.

For Sarah, aiming to improve her family's health and expand her knowledge of diets, the low-FODMAP diet offers a universe of benefits. As a culinary adventure, it could introduce her and her family to a world of new, exciting foods they might not have considered before. Sarah could turn the challenge of managing FODMAPs into a delightful exploration of varied cuisines and unique ingredients.

The low-FODMAP diet also encourages cooking at home, creating an opportunity for quality family time. Preparing meals together could become an engaging educational experience for her children, instilling in them an appreciation for wholesome, nutritious food from a young age. It's more than just about eating right; it's about cultivating a healthier relationship with food.

The benefits extend to Sarah's professional growth as well. By delving into the intricacies of the low-FODMAP diet, she'd gain a more profound understanding of nutrition and dietary impacts on health, enhancing her career prospects in the health and wellness field.

Lastly, the relief from IBS symptoms could alleviate social anxiety linked to dining out. Both Mike and Sarah could find themselves more at ease in social settings, no longer worrying about the immediate after-effects of meals. They could savor their moments, whether during a high-powered business lunch or a laid-back family dinner, without the looming fear of an IBS flare-up.

In essence, the lifestyle benefits of a low-FODMAP diet extend beyond the realm of physical health. It branches into the realms of mental well-being, social ease, familial bonds, and personal and professional development, painting a holistic picture of improved life quality.

Your Guide Through The Cookbook: Exploring A New Culinary Journey

Embarking on a new dietary plan can often feel daunting, but it needn't be so with this cookbook in your hands. Consider this cookbook your companion and guide, an enthusiastic cheerleader, and a patient teacher as you set off on your low-FODMAP adventure.

Now, Mike, our fitness enthusiast battling IBS, might be wondering, "How can this cookbook help me manage my symptoms and maintain my fitness level?" And Sarah, our health-conscious mom and ambitious career woman, might be pondering, "How can this cookbook improve my family's health and boost my understanding of diverse diets?" This cookbook is here to answer those questions.

Each recipe in this cookbook has been crafted with you in mind. Every dish is not just a meal but a step toward achieving your goals. For Mike, it's about creating meals that are easy on the gut, but can fuel a strenuous workout. For Sarah, it's about providing wholesome, nutritious food for her family that doesn't sacrifice taste for health.

The recipes in this book span a variety of culinary traditions, showcasing the diversity of a low-FODMAP diet. It shatters the misconception that dietary restrictions limit food choices. Instead, this cookbook expands your culinary horizons, exposing you to a myriad of flavors and textures, while respecting the principles of a low-FODMAP diet.

It's not just about what you can or cannot eat, but also about learning new cooking techniques, and how to substitute high-FODMAP ingredients with low-FODMAP alternatives. This cookbook serves as a culinary education, broadening your understanding of food and nutrition. For Sarah, it might even become a cornerstone resource in her professional life.

Moreover, this cookbook does not merely hand you a list of recipes. It is designed to educate you on why certain ingredients are used, their health benefits, and how they fit into a low-FODMAP diet. It empowers you to make informed decisions about your food, fostering a deeper connection between you and your meals. It inspires creativity, giving you the confidence to experiment and adapt the recipes to your preferences.

This cookbook appreciates that you lead a busy life. It respects that time is a luxury. That's why you'll find the recipes organized by their prep and cooking times, helping you plan your meals efficiently. Quick breakfast options for rushed mornings, leisurely brunch recipes for lazy weekends, and easy dinner solutions for busy weeknights—this cookbook has it all.

Whether you are well-versed in the kitchen or a cooking novice, whether you are a foodie who loves to explore or someone who sticks to classics, this cookbook welcomes you. It's more than just a collection of low-FODMAP recipes; it's a guide, a teacher, and a friend on your journey toward a healthier, more comfortable life. So, let's flip the page and start this new culinary journey together.

Finding Your Way Through the Recipes: A Path to Culinary Success

As you journey into the world of low-FODMAP cuisine, you might wonder how to navigate through the multitude of recipes included in this cookbook. The array of dishes may seem overwhelming initially, but rest assured, this book is designed to guide you smoothly through your culinary expedition.

To ensure an enriching and enjoyable experience, the cookbook's design focuses on user-friendly navigation. The purpose is to accommodate your lifestyle, your pace, and your learning curve, making it as effortless as possible for both Mike, our fitness-loving IBS warrior, and Sarah, our health-conscious mom and career woman.

Every recipe in this cookbook begins with a brief introduction. This isn't merely a way to present the dish but a window into its character, significance, and how it can contribute to your low-FODMAP journey. It provides you a context, a story, and most importantly, a connection to the food you will prepare.

Each recipe is then outlined in a step-by-step manner. The instructions are clear, precise, and devoid of culinary jargon that could mystify a novice. The aim is to make every cooking step feel like a comfortable conversation rather than a stiff lecture, ensuring that both the seasoned cook and the kitchen newbie feel equally at home.

Every recipe also includes preparation and cooking time. This feature allows you to choose dishes that align with your schedule, making meal planning less of a chore and more of a delight. Need a quick, nutritious breakfast before heading to the gym, Mike? Or a healthy, easy-to-prepare dinner that will delight your family, Sarah? The times listed with each recipe will help guide your choices.

Ingredients are another vital aspect. The recipes include common, easy-to-find ingredients, ensuring that adhering to a low-FODMAP diet doesn't mean hunting for obscure items at specialty stores. Additionally, each ingredient is annotated with its FODMAP content, guiding you through the process and assisting you in managing your intake.

To cater to your diverse needs, the cookbook also features a variety of recipes, each labeled by meal type, cuisine, and even occasions. You'll find dishes for breakfast, lunch, dinner, and those in-between snacks. From comfort foods and festive fare to quick bites and gourmet meals, the recipes are as diverse as your own tastes and requirements.

Finally, the recipes are not static; they are adaptable. Each one comes with suggestions for variations, making them flexible to your taste preferences or dietary requirements. Think of these recipes as a base, a starting point, from which you can explore and experiment, guided by your palate.

The goal of this cookbook is not to dictate your meals but to inspire, empower, and guide you through your low-FODMAP journey. The intention is to make your transition to this lifestyle not just manageable, but also enjoyable, turning each recipe into a delightful culinary adventure. So flip the page, pick a recipe that speaks to you, and let's begin this delicious journey together.

Charting Your Course: A Guide to the Meal Plan

Now, you've come to the part of the book where it all comes together - the meal plan. Consider this the map for your journey into the low-FODMAP lifestyle. We have done the hard work of collating the recipes into a guide that can cater to your weekly needs, fitting seamlessly into the rhythm of your everyday life.

Why a meal plan? Because it's the compass that will steer your dietary choices, guiding you in maintaining balance in FODMAP intake throughout the day, and the week. This tool will help you avoid the pitfalls of high-FODMAP foods while enjoying a variety of low-FODMAP dishes.

When you glance at the meal plan, you'll notice it's not just a random assortment of recipes. Instead, it's a careful orchestration of meals. Let's walk through how it works.

The meal plan is laid out weekly, with each day broken down into breakfast, lunch, dinner, and two snacks. This structure ensures you have a sustained supply of energy throughout the day. For Mike, who is juggling a demanding career with his fitness goals, this could mean the difference between a productive day and a day of feeling drained. For Sarah, who's committed to nourishing her family with wholesome meals, this organization ensures she always knows what's on the menu, relieving her from the stress of daily meal planning.

Each day's meals are thoughtfully combined to offer a range of nutrients and variety in flavors, making sure your diet is balanced, your palate is entertained, and most importantly, your intake of FODMAPs remains within recommended levels.

The meal plan also considers practicality. Busy days are complemented with meals that are quick and easy to prepare, while more relaxed times may feature dishes that involve a little more time in the kitchen, turning meal preparation into a joyful culinary adventure rather than a race against time.

Another feature of the meal plan is its adaptability. It's not set in stone, but designed to be flexible, respecting your individual preferences and needs. We've suggested alternatives for some meals and snacks, accommodating different tastes and dietary requirements.

Moreover, the meal plan accounts for leftovers. We know how valuable your time is. By strategically incorporating meals that yield more than one serving, you can cook once and eat twice, or even thrice, saving your valuable time without compromising on the quality of your meals.

Finally, the meal plan is more than a chart of what to eat and when. It's a resource to learn, explore, and master the low-FODMAP lifestyle. By following the meal plan, you'll cultivate an intuitive understanding of combining foods and managing your FODMAP intake. This skill will empower you to gradually design your own meal plans, turning the low-FODMAP diet into a sustainable lifestyle.

So, dive into the meal plan with an open mind. Use it as a guide, not a mandate. Embrace its flexibility, enjoy the variety, and most importantly, savor the journey into a healthier, more comfortable, and flavorful life.

We've reached the end of this enlightening chapter where we've unpacked FODMAP, illuminated its relationship with IBS, and investigated how a low-FODMAP diet can trigger positive health transformations and lifestyle adjustments. The rewards of this dietary approach, supported by scientific research, create a promising panorama for those ready to embark on this journey.

Equipped with this cookbook and a comprehensive meal plan, your transition into a low-FODMAP lifestyle becomes more straightforward. With these tools, you can adapt to your unique tastes and needs. As you dive into the cookbook and adapt to the meal plan, you'll find yourself gradually mastering the art of combining foods and balancing your FODMAP intake.

Armed with this newfound knowledge and handy tools, you're prepared to set sail on your low-FODMAP journey. Remember, this journey is about nurturing a healthier bond with food and reveling in the process as much as the results. As you turn the leaf to the upcoming chapter, bear in mind that each minor change cascades into a larger transformation. So, let's embark on this exciting journey together!

Chapter 2: Getting Started

Embarking on the journey of a low-FODMAP diet can feel like navigating uncharted waters. There's so much to learn, so many things to consider. This journey, however, is not about confining your culinary experiences. On the contrary, it opens up a new world of flavors, textures, and cooking adventures. Chapter 2, "Getting Started", aims to guide you as you prepare for this exciting exploration of low-FODMAP cuisine. From preparing your kitchen, identifying and sourcing essential ingredients, to mastering the art of reading labels and substituting high-FODMAP ingredients, we will navigate these new territories together. Whether your goal is to manage IBS symptoms, maintain fitness, or improve family health while expanding dietary knowledge, this chapter equips you with practical tools to confidently step into your low-FODMAP culinary adventure.

Preparing Your Kitchen for a Low-FODMAP Diet

Setting off on the low-FODMAP journey is akin to embarking on a new adventure. And like every well-planned adventure, your journey too begins at home, more specifically, in the heart of your home—the kitchen.

Cleaning Out the Pantry

The transition to a low-FODMAP diet entails understanding that not all food items you used to love can accompany you on this journey. It's akin to outgrowing old habits and welcoming new ones that serve you better. And the first tangible step towards that is cleaning out your pantry.

Just as you would organize your workspace before starting an important project, arranging your pantry can help you embark on this low-FODMAP journey with a clear mind and a definite direction. Start by taking out all the items and setting them on your kitchen counter. Check the labels for high-FODMAP ingredients—think wheat, lactose, certain fruits like apples and pears, and specific vegetables such as onions and garlic.

It's a meticulous process, but one that's essential in paving the way for a pantry that aligns with your dietary goals. Remember, it isn't about depriving yourself but about replacing high-FODMAP items with alternatives that are just as delectable yet much friendlier to your gut.

Essential Kitchen Tools

Having the right tools is as crucial in the kitchen as it is in any craft. As you delve into low-FODMAP cooking, certain tools can make your culinary journey a breeze.

First, let's talk about storage. Proper containers are essential for keeping your low-FODMAP ingredients fresh and preventing cross-contamination. Glass containers with airtight lids are an excellent option—they're durable, environmentally friendly, and don't harbor food smells.

A slow cooker is another worthwhile investment. With your busy urban lifestyle, it's an appliance that can make cooking low-FODMAP meals easy and convenient. Imagine Mike, coming home from an intense workout, to a slow-cooked, low-FODMAP chili that's been simmering all day—nourishing, comforting, and gentle on his gut.

Don't underestimate the power of a quality set of knives. Precision in chopping can affect cooking times and even the release of FODMAPs in some foods.

Then, there's the humble blender, an unsung hero in the low-FODMAP kitchen. A quick whirl, and you can have everything from green smoothies and pureed soups to homemade sauces free of garlic and onions—dishes that Sarah, on a mission to improve her family's health, would be eager to add to her repertoire.

So, outfitting your kitchen for your low-FODMAP journey doesn't mean investing in the latest fancy gadgets. Instead, it involves mindful selection of tools that align with your dietary goals and fit seamlessly into your lifestyle, making the process of cooking and eating enjoyable, effortless, and most importantly, conducive to health and well-being.

Essential Low-FODMAP Ingredients

While the cornerstone of the low-FODMAP diet is about knowing what to avoid, it's equally vital to know what you should fill your shopping cart with. Having an arsenal of low-FODMAP ingredients can transform your culinary experience from a restrictive diet plan to an exciting culinary exploration.

Pantry Staples

The backbone of any kitchen, pantry staples, are the essentials that shape your day-to-day cooking. Embracing a low-FODMAP lifestyle means modifying this list to be gut-friendly yet as tantalizing to your taste buds as ever.

Start with grains. Rice, oats, and quinoa are your new best friends. They are versatile, satiating, and most importantly, low in FODMAPs. For Mike, who aims to maintain his fitness levels, these complex carbohydrates can provide a sustained energy release throughout his workout routines.

Consider investing in gluten-free flours like rice flour or almond flour for your baking needs. But remember, gluten-free doesn't always translate to low-FODMAP. It's always a good idea to read the labels for any hidden high-FODMAP ingredients.

Next, let's address the elephant in the room—dairy. Lactose-free milk and hard cheeses like cheddar or swiss are generally well-tolerated. You could also explore dairy alternatives like almond milk or coconut yogurt.

Spices and condiments can make or break a dish. Rest assured, there are plenty of low-FODMAP options—garlic-infused oils for the much-needed aroma, tamari sauce as a soy sauce substitute, and a range of herbs and spices to make your meals flavorful and exciting.

Fresh Produce

The world of fresh produce on a low-FODMAP diet is colorful and varied. Sarah, eager to better her family's health through diet, would be glad to know that there's a rainbow of fruits and vegetables that are low in FODMAPs.

Start with leafy greens—spinach, kale, lettuce, the list is quite extensive. Not only are they low in FODMAPs, but they're also chock-full of vitamins and minerals. Root vegetables like potatoes and carrots are excellent options too. They're hearty, versatile, and provide a comforting familiarity in your culinary endeavors.

Fruits can be a tricky area, but once you know what to choose, they can add a delightful freshness to your meals. Blueberries, strawberries, oranges, and grapes are some of the low-FODMAP fruits that can bring a burst of flavors to your breakfast cereals or afternoon snacks.

Proteins

Protein sources, for the most part, are low in FODMAPs, making them a key component of your diet. Whether you're a meat-eater, vegetarian, or vegan, there are plenty of options to meet your protein needs.

Chicken, fish, beef, or eggs can easily find a place in your low-FODMAP meal plans. For our vegetarian and vegan friends, options like tempeh and firm tofu can provide the much-needed protein content.

Remember, it's not just about the kind of protein but also how it's prepared. Try to avoid marinades and sauces that could contain high-FODMAP ingredients. Sometimes, simplicity is key—a dash of salt, a squeeze of lemon, and a sprinkle of herbs can go a long way.

Incorporating these low-FODMAP ingredients in your pantry, fridge, and meal plans can provide a solid foundation for your dietary journey. With the right ingredients, not only can you manage your IBS symptoms effectively, but also discover a whole new world of flavors and textures, making your meals anything but monotonous. Your health goals don't have to be a compromise on your taste buds, and these ingredients are proof of that.

Tips for Shopping and Reading Labels

Starting on the low-FODMAP diet path can be compared to becoming a food detective of sorts. You'll need to learn how to decipher food labels, ensuring that what you consume won't exacerbate your IBS symptoms. Don't be daunted by this task, though; it's empowering to know what you're putting in your body. Knowledge, after all, is power.

Identifying High-FODMAP Ingredients

To transition to a low-FODMAP diet, you must become adept at identifying high-FODMAP ingredients. These are not your enemies—rather, they're just foods that your gut finds more challenging to digest. Typical high-FODMAP ingredients to look out for include wheat, onions, garlic, high fructose corn syrup, and some fruits and vegetables. However, they can often be disguised under different names. For instance, wheat might be listed as flour, bread crumbs, or semolina. Meanwhile, fructose might hide behind the names of agave nectar or fruit juice concentrate.

Other ingredients that are high in FODMAPs include chicory root, inulin, or anything labeled as 'fructooligosaccharides' or 'FOS.' Also, sugar-free or diet products often contain sweeteners like sorbitol, mannitol, and xylitol, which are high in FODMAPs.

The list might seem overwhelming initially, but remember, this journey is a learning curve. As you familiarize yourself with high-FODMAP ingredients and their aliases, you'll soon spot them with ease.

Shopping Tips

Successfully shopping for a low-FODMAP diet requires a few savvy strategies. These will make your grocery shopping less of a chore and more of an empowering experience.

Firstly, planning is crucial. By planning your meals and writing a grocery list, you save time, reduce stress, and maintain focus during your shopping trip.

Secondly, knowing your stores is a game-changer. Each grocery store varies, and some will offer a better selection of low-FODMAP foods than others. Mike, living in an urban area, might find local health food stores, international markets, or even online retailers that cater to his dietary needs.

Prioritizing fresh produce and proteins is another effective strategy. These food items are naturally low in FODMAPs and are devoid of any additives or hidden ingredients. Sarah, aiming to enhance her family's health, can depend on fresh foods for their natural flavors and nutritious benefits.

However, don't discount the freezer section. Frozen fruits and vegetables are excellent low-FODMAP options. They are as nutritious as fresh ones and provide convenience and variety.

When in the grocery store, it is usually best to stick to the perimeter. This is where fresh foods are typically located, while processed foods fill the middle aisles. This tactic helps you focus on low-FODMAP foods.

Being label-savvy is another crucial skill. It's essential to stay vigilant about high-FODMAP ingredients. At the same time, other nutritional aspects like sodium, sugar, and fat content should not be overlooked.

Lastly, embrace the opportunity to try new foods. The low-FODMAP diet can expand your palate, and who knows, you might discover a new favorite dish.

By employing these strategies, shopping for a low-FODMAP diet will become less of a challenge and more of a joy. Remember, the goal is to make mindful choices that cater to your dietary needs without compromising on taste or nutritional value. This approach can offer immense benefits to Sarah, who wants to expand her knowledge of diets, and to Mike, who aims to manage his IBS symptoms, making them savvy shoppers and skilled label readers.

Substituting High-FODMAP Ingredients

Taking on a low-FODMAP diet does not necessitate bidding farewell to all your favorite dishes. In fact, this new dietary regimen opens the door to a world of culinary exploration. The key to unlocking this door lies in learning how to substitute high-FODMAP ingredients with their low-FODMAP counterparts. Let's delve into the most common substitutions and a few creative swaps you can make.

Common Substitutions

For a lot of staple foods that are high in FODMAPs, there are readily available alternatives that are equally tasty and far easier on your digestive system. For instance, wheat products such as bread, pasta, and pastries, are high in FODMAPs. But that doesn't mean you have to let go of these comfort foods. Instead, you can substitute them with products made from gluten-free grains like rice, quinoa, or buckwheat.

Other examples of easy swaps include replacing cow's milk with lactose-free milk or plant-based milks like almond or rice milk. Instead of using onions and garlic to flavor your meals, you can use the green parts of spring onions and leeks, and garlic-infused oil which are all low in FODMAPs.

A common misconception is that a low-FODMAP diet is restrictive. This is far from the truth. Mike, who is keen on maintaining his fitness level, can still enjoy a wide variety of foods that provide all the necessary nutrients, while Sarah can prepare wholesome and delicious meals that align with the family's health goals.

Creative Swaps

There's a world of culinary opportunities when you think creatively. Instead of viewing the low-FODMAP diet as a list of 'can't haves,' view it as an invitation to discover new ingredients and flavors.

For example, when it comes to fruits, apples and pears might be off-limits due to their high FODMAP content, but there are numerous other options like blueberries, grapes, and pineapples. You can even get adventurous and try more exotic fruits like dragon fruit or starfruit, if they're available in your area.

Let's consider sweeteners. Honey and agave syrup are high in FODMAPs, but that doesn't mean you can't enjoy the sweetness in your life. Maple syrup and rice malt syrup are excellent alternatives. Or perhaps you'd like to experiment with coconut sugar or date syrup for a touch of the exotic.

For individuals like Sarah, who are looking to expand their diet knowledge for their career, experimenting with these creative swaps can add an extra layer of expertise. She can showcase a range of recipes that not only adhere to low-FODMAP guidelines but also introduce a global palate to her clientele.

Substituting high-FODMAP ingredients doesn't necessarily mean compromising on taste or diversity in your diet. The low-FODMAP diet is a journey of discovery. With every new ingredient you find, you'll be one step closer to transforming your relationship with food and taking control of your health. Remember, the low-FODMAP diet is not a life sentence, but rather a management tool, a means to understand your triggers and work towards a happier, healthier you. For Mike, this means managing his IBS symptoms, and for Sarah, it means improving her family's health while advancing her career. The power of food is truly remarkable, and a low-FODMAP diet is a testament to this.

Taking the first steps toward embracing a low-FODMAP diet can be challenging. The transition may seem complex, and the task of replacing familiar ingredients daunting. However, with the knowledge gained in this chapter, you now have the power to transform your kitchen and your eating habits. By preparing your kitchen, learning about essential low-FODMAP ingredients, shopping smartly, and mastering substitutions, you're well-equipped to succeed in your low-FODMAP journey. This is not merely a diet. It's a lifestyle change that has the potential to drastically improve your health and quality of life. Remember, your effort in adopting this new way of eating is an investment in your future health and wellbeing. Let's continue to explore and appreciate the remarkable power of food together in the coming chapters.

Chapter 3: Breakfast Recipes

1. Introduction to Breakfast

In this chapter, we'll redefine breakfast from the perspective of a Low-FODMAP diet. We'll introduce recipes that are not just about feeding morning hunger but also about addressing gut health. The range includes quick 20-minute meals for the busy bees and more indulgent, elaborate ones for leisurely mornings. We have both light and hearty options to cater to various preferences.

Embracing a Low-FODMAP breakfast isn't about limiting your choices. On the contrary, it's an opportunity to explore new ingredients and unique combinations. Each recipe is a step towards better digestive health without compromising on taste.

So, buckle up for this flavorful journey of Low-FODMAP breakfast recipes. Let's transform your mornings into a delightful culinary experience that is also kind to your gut. Whether you're a breakfast enthusiast or just beginning to establish a morning meal routine, this chapter promises something for everyone.

Detailed recipes

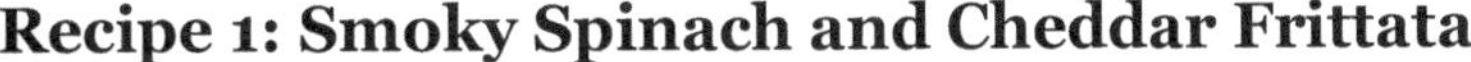

Recipe 1: Smoky Spinach and Cheddar Frittata

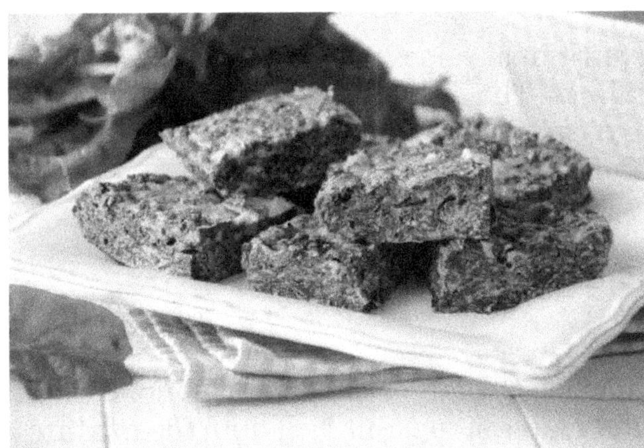

P. T. : 10 minutes
C. T. : 20 minutes
Ingr. :
- 6 eggs
- 1/4 cup lactose-free milk
- 1 cup cheddar cheese
- 2 cups spinach
- 1 teaspoon smoked paprika
- Salt and pepper to taste

Serv. : 4
M. of C. : Oven-baked
Procedure:
Whisk eggs with lactose-free milk, smoked paprika, salt, and pepper. Stir in cheese and spinach. Pour into a greased baking dish and bake at 375°F (190°C) for 20 minutes or until set.
N. V. :
Approximately 250 calories, 20g protein, 3g carbohydrates, 18g fat per serving.

Recipe 2: Low-FODMAP Peanut Butter & Banana Oatmeal

P. T. : 5 minutes
C. T. : 10 minutes
Ingr. :

- 1 cup gluten-free oats
- 2 cups water
- A pinch of salt
- 2 tablespoons peanut butter
- 1 medium ripe banana, sliced

Serv. : 2
M. of C. : Stovetop

Procedure:
Combine oats, water, and a pinch of salt in a saucepan. Bring to a boil, then reduce heat and simmer, stirring occasionally, for 10 minutes or until oats are your desired thickness. Stir in peanut butter until well combined. Serve with banana slices on top.
N. V. :
Approximately 350 calories, 11g protein, 55g carbohydrates, 11g fat per serving.

Recipe 3: Savory Buckwheat Crepes

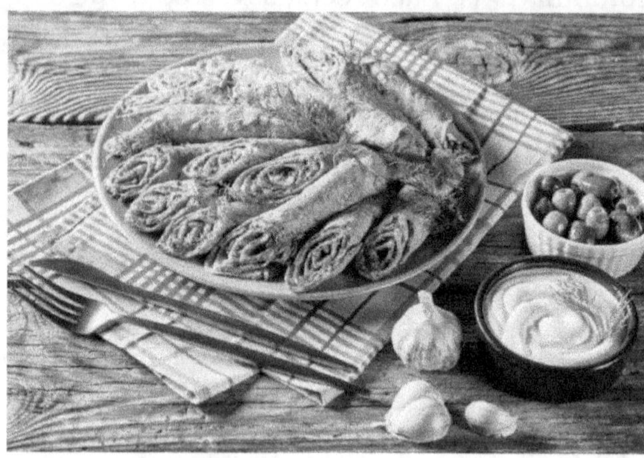

P. T. : 20 minutes
C. T. : 30 minutes
Ingr. :

- 1 cup buckwheat flour
- 2 large eggs
- 1 1/4 cups lactose-free milk
- Pinch of salt
- 2 tablespoons olive oil
- Fillings of choice (grilled vegetables, ham, cheese)

Serv. : 4
M. of C. : Pan-frying
Procedure:
In a large bowl, mix together buckwheat flour, eggs, milk, and salt until smooth. Heat a crepe pan or large skillet over medium heat and brush with olive oil. Pour 1/4 of the batter into the pan, swirling to fully cover the surface. Cook until golden brown on both sides, flipping once. Repeat with remaining batter. Fill crepes with your choice of fillings.
N. V. :
Nutritional values will vary depending on fillings. The base crepe has approximately 150 calories, 7g protein, 20g carbohydrates, and 5g fat per serving.

Recipe 4: Chia Seed Pudding

P. T. : 10 minutes
Resting Time: 2 hours
Ingr. :

- ¼ cup chia seeds
- 1 cup almond milk, unsweetened
- 1 tablespoon pure maple syrup
- Toppings: A small handful of blueberries and strawberries

Serv. : 2
M. of C. : Refrigeration

Procedure:
In a bowl, combine chia seeds, almond milk, and maple syrup. Stir well until the mixture starts to thicken. Cover and set in the refrigerator for at least 2 hours or overnight. The chia seeds will absorb the liquid and grow in size, resulting in a pudding-like consistency. Serve cold with a handful of blueberries and strawberries on top.
N. V. :

Approximately 150 calories, 4g protein, 20g carbohydrates, and 6g fat per serving.

Recipe 5: Scrambled Tofu with Spinach and Bell Peppers

P. T. : 10 minutes
C. T. : 15 minutes
Ingr. :

- 1 block (14 oz) firm tofu, drained and crumbled
- 1 cup fresh spinach
- 1 bell pepper, diced
- 2 tablespoons olive oil
- Salt and pepper to taste

Serv. : 4
M. of C. : Pan-frying

Procedure:
Heat the olive oil in a skillet over medium heat. Add the bell pepper and sauté until it starts to soften. Add the crumbled tofu and cook for a few minutes, stirring frequently. Lastly, add the fresh spinach and cook until wilted. Season with salt and pepper to taste.

N. V. :
Approximately 150 calories, 11g protein, 6g carbohydrates, and 10g fat per serving.

Recipe 6: Low-FODMAP Oatmeal

P. T. : 2 minutes
C. T. : 10 minutes
Ingr. :

- 1 cup gluten-free oats
- 2 cups almond milk
- A pinch of salt
- 1 tablespoon maple syrup
- Toppings: A small handful of blueberries and sliced almonds

Serv. : 2
M. of C. : Stovetop boiling
Procedure:

Combine the oats and almond milk in a saucepan over medium heat. Add a pinch of salt. Cook the mixture, stirring occasionally, until the oats have absorbed the liquid and are creamy. This should take about 10 minutes. Once cooked, sweeten your oatmeal with some maple syrup. Serve warm and top with a handful of blueberries and some sliced almonds for extra crunch.

N. V. :
Approximately 210 calories, 6g protein, 36g carbohydrates, and 6g fat per serving.

Recipe 7: Quinoa Porridge with Berries

P. T. : 5 minutes
C. T. : 15 minutes
Ingr. :

- 1/2 cup uncooked quinoa
- 1 cup almond milk
- 1/2 cup water
- 1 tablespoon maple syrup
- Toppings: A small handful of blueberries and strawberries

Serv. : 2
M. of C. : Stovetop boiling
Procedure:

First, rinse the quinoa under cold water until the water runs clear. Combine the rinsed quinoa, almond milk, and water in a saucepan. Bring the mixture to a boil over medium-high heat. Once boiling, reduce the heat to low and let it simmer for about 15 minutes, or until the quinoa is tender and the liquid is absorbed. Sweeten your porridge with maple syrup and top with a small handful of fresh berries.

N. V. :
Approximately 220 calories, 8g protein, 40g carbohydrates, and 3.5g fat per serving.

Recipe 8: Avocado and Tomato on Gluten-free Toast

P. T. : 5 minutes
C. T. : 5 minutes
Ingr. :
- 2 slices of gluten-free bread
- 1 ripe avocado
- A handful of cherry tomatoes
- Salt and pepper to taste

Serv. : 2
M. of C. : Toasting and assembly
Procedure:

First, toast the gluten-free bread to your desired crispness. In the meantime, slice the avocado and cherry tomatoes. Once the toast is ready, top each slice with the sliced avocado and tomatoes. Season with salt and pepper to taste.

N. V. :
Approximately 210 calories, 4g protein, 24g carbohydrates, and 11g fat per serving.

Recipe 9: Scrambled Tofu with Spinach

P. T. : 5 minutes
C. T. : 10 minutes
Ingr. :
- 1/2 block firm tofu
- 2 cups fresh spinach
- 1/4 teaspoon turmeric
- 1/4 teaspoon cumin
- Salt and pepper to taste
- 1 tablespoon olive oil

Serv. : 2
M. of C. : Sauté
Procedure:

First, press the tofu to remove excess water and crumble it into small pieces. Heat the olive oil in a non-stick pan over medium heat. Add the crumbled tofu, turmeric, and cumin to the pan and stir well to evenly distribute the spices. Sauté the tofu until it starts to turn golden brown. Add the fresh spinach and continue cooking until the spinach wilts. Season with salt and pepper to taste.

N. V. :
Approximately 150 calories, 13g protein, 6g carbohydrates, and 9g fat per serving.

Recipe 10: Banana Pancakes with Blueberries

P. T. : 10 minutes
C. T. : 15 minutes
Ingr. :
- 1 ripe banana
- 2 eggs
- 1/2 cup gluten-free oats
- 1/4 teaspoon baking powder
- A handful of blueberries
- 1 tablespoon maple syrup

Serv. : 2
M. of C. : Blending and pan-frying
Procedure:

In a blender, combine the ripe banana, eggs, gluten-free oats, and baking powder. Blend until you get a smooth batter. Heat a non-stick pan over medium heat. Pour 1/4 cup of the batter into the pan for each pancake. Add a few blueberries on top of each pancake before flipping. Cook until golden brown on both sides. Serve with a drizzle of maple syrup.

N. V. :
Approximately 290 calories, 11g protein, 51g carbohydrates, and 7g fat per serving.

Recipe 11: Egg and Spinach Frittata

P. T. : 10 minutes
C. T. : 20 minutes

Ingr. :
- 6 eggs

- 2 cups fresh spinach
- 1/2 cup diced bell pepper
- Salt and pepper to taste
- 1 tablespoon olive oil

Serv. : 4
M. of C. : Sauté and oven-bake
Procedure:
Preheat your oven to 350°F (175°C). In a bowl, beat the eggs and season with salt and pepper. Heat the olive oil in an oven-safe skillet over medium heat. Add the diced bell pepper and sauté until tender. Add the spinach and cook until wilted. Pour the beaten eggs over the vegetables and stir gently to combine. Transfer the skillet to the preheated oven and bake for 20 minutes, or until the eggs are set.
N. V. :
Approximately 150 calories, 12g protein, 3g carbohydrates, and 10g fat per serving.

Recipe 12: Quinoa Porridge with Mixed Berries

P. T. : 10 minutes
C. T. : 20 minutes
Ingr. :
- 1/2 cup uncooked quinoa
- 1 cup almond milk
- 1 tablespoon maple syrup
- 1/2 teaspoon vanilla extract
- 1 cup mixed berries

Serv. : 2
M. of C. : Simmer
Procedure:
Rinse the quinoa under cold water to remove any saponin coating. Place the quinoa and almond milk in a saucepan and bring it to a boil. Reduce the heat and let it simmer for 15-20 minutes, or until the quinoa is tender and the liquid is absorbed. Stir in the maple syrup and vanilla extract. Serve the porridge with a topping of mixed berries.
N. V. :
Approximately 240 calories, 8g protein, 43g carbohydrates, and 5g fat per serving.

Recipe 13: Buckwheat Pancakes with Maple Syrup

P. T. : 10 minutes
C. T. : 15 minutes
Ingr. :
- 1 cup buckwheat flour
- 1 teaspoon baking powder
- 1 tablespoon maple syrup
- 1 cup almond milk
- 1 egg
- Salt to taste

Serv. : 4
M. of C. : Pan-frying
Procedure:
In a bowl, mix the buckwheat flour, baking powder, and a pinch of salt. In another bowl, whisk the egg, almond milk, and maple syrup together. Gradually add the wet ingredients to the dry ingredients and stir until you get a smooth batter. Heat a non-stick pan over medium heat. Pour 1/4 cup of the batter into the pan for each pancake. Cook until bubbles appear on the surface, then flip and cook until golden brown. Serve with a drizzle of maple syrup.
N. V. :
Approximately 200 calories, 7g protein, 38g carbohydrates, and 3g fat per serving.

Recipe 14: Chia Seed Pudding with Kiwi and Coconut

P. T. : 5 minutes
Resting Time: Overnight
Ingr. :
- 3 tablespoons chia seeds
- 1 cup almond milk
- 1 tablespoon maple syrup
- 1 kiwi, sliced
- 1 tablespoon shredded coconut

Serv. : 1
M. of C. : No-cook, resting
Procedure:
In a bowl or a mason jar, combine the chia seeds, almond milk, and maple syrup. Stir well to avoid any clumps. Let the mixture rest in the fridge overnight. In the morning, stir the pudding and top it with sliced kiwi and shredded coconut.
N. V. :
Approximately 350 calories, 11g protein, 45g carbohydrates, and 15g fat per serving.

Recipe 15: Banana and Walnut Muffins

P. T. : 15 minutes
C. T. : 25 minutes
Ingr. :
- 1 ripe banana, mashed
- 1/2 cup almond flour
- 2 eggs
- 1/4 cup walnuts, chopped
- 1 tablespoon maple syrup
- 1/2 teaspoon baking powder
- Pinch of salt

Serv. : 6
M. of C. : Baking
Procedure:
Preheat your oven to 350°F (175°C). In a bowl, combine the almond flour, baking powder, and salt. In another bowl, whisk the eggs and add the mashed banana and maple syrup. Gradually add the dry ingredients to the wet ones and stir until well combined. Fold in the chopped walnuts. Pour the mixture into muffin cups, filling each one two-thirds of the way. Bake for 25 minutes or until a toothpick comes out clean.
N. V. :
Approximately 140 calories, 5g protein, 12g carbohydrates, and 9g fat per serving.

Recipe 16: Omelet with Spinach and Feta Cheese

P. T. : 10 minutes
C. T. : 10 minutes
Ingr. :
- 2 eggs
- 1/2 cup spinach, chopped
- 2 tablespoons feta cheese, crumbled
- Salt and pepper to taste
- 1 teaspoon olive oil

Serv. : 1
M. of C. : Pan-frying
Procedure:
In a bowl, beat the eggs and season with salt and pepper. Heat the olive oil in a non-stick pan over medium heat. Add the chopped spinach and sauté until wilted. Pour the beaten eggs over the spinach and cook until almost set. Sprinkle the crumbled feta cheese on top and fold the omelet in half. Cook for another minute, then serve.
N. V. :
Approximately 240 calories, 14g protein, 2g carbohydrates, and 18g fat per serving

Recipe 17: Smoothie Bowl with Berries and Chia Seeds

P. T. : 5 minutes
C. T. : None
Ingr. :
- 1/2 cup mixed berries
- 1 ripe banana
- 1/2 cup almond milk
- 1 tablespoon chia seeds
- 1 tablespoon coconut flakes

Serv. : 1
M. of C. : Blending
Procedure:
In a blender, combine the mixed berries, banana, and almond milk until smooth. Pour the mixture into a bowl. Top with chia seeds and coconut flakes, and serve.
N. V. :

Approximately 320 calories, 8g protein, 53g carbohydrates, and 11g fat per serving.

Recipe 18: Granola with Almonds and Dried Fruit

P. T. : 10 minutes
C. T. : 20 minutes
Ingr. :
- 2 cups rolled oats
- 1/2 cup almonds, chopped
- 1/4 cup dried fruit, chopped
- 2 tablespoons maple syrup
- 1 tablespoon coconut oil

Serv. : 8
M. of C. : Baking
Procedure:

Preheat your oven to 300°F (150°C). In a bowl, mix the rolled oats and chopped almonds. In a small saucepan, melt the coconut oil and maple syrup together, then pour over the oats and almonds. Stir well to combine. Spread the mixture on a baking sheet and bake for 20 minutes or until golden brown. Let it cool, then stir in the dried fruit.

N. V. :
Approximately 200 calories, 6g protein, 28g carbohydrates, and 8g fat per serving.

Chapter 4: Lunch Recipes

Introduction to Lunch

Welcome to the exciting world of lunchtime recipes on a Low-FODMAP diet. This midday meal is a perfect balance between necessity and enjoyment, carrying its own uniqueness, neither as predictable as breakfast nor as experimental as dinner. For the diligent men managing IBS and maintaining fitness, and the health-conscious women seeking dietary knowledge for family health and professional growth, lunchtime is an essential player.

A Low-FODMAP diet aims to reduce certain sugars that could trigger gut-related symptoms, but that doesn't mean monotony. The recipes we present here, from salads and soups to proteins and veggies, will show you the delightful diversity achievable within this dietary regimen.

Embrace lunch as a moment of calm in your bustling day. Step away from your workspace, engage with your food, appreciate its flavors, and the nourishment it provides. This is crucial for maintaining good gut health.

The recipes will introduce a variety of ingredients, some familiar, some new. Do not fear the unknown. In food, unfamiliarity is a chance to expand your culinary scope. We hope that you'll start to anticipate lunch, not as a hurried necessity but as a key part of your daily wellness routine.

So, get your cooking tools ready, and let's transform lunch from an ordinary meal into an extraordinary health and taste experience. Happy cooking!

Detailed recipes

Recipe 1: Low-FODMAP Lemon Chicken Salad

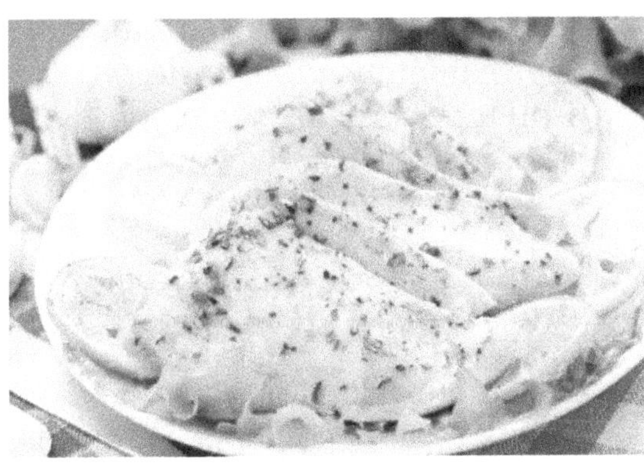

- **P. T. :** 20 minutes
- **Ingr. :** 2 skinless chicken breasts, 1 tablespoon of garlic-infused oil, 2 tablespoons of lemon juice, 1 teaspoon of dried basil, salt and pepper to taste, 2 cups of mixed salad greens, 1 sliced cucumber, 10 cherry tomatoes, 1/2 cup of sliced black olives
- **Servings :** Serves 2
- **M. of C. :** Grilling

- **Process:** Marinate the chicken breasts in the garlic-infused oil, lemon juice, basil, salt, and pepper for at least 15 minutes. Grill the chicken until fully cooked and allow to cool. Slice the cooked chicken and toss with the salad greens, cucumber, tomatoes, and olives. Drizzle with extra lemon juice and garlic-infused oil if desired.
- **N. V. :** Each serving contains approximately 320 calories, 30g of protein, 14g of fat, 20g of carbohydrates, and 5g of fiber.

Recipe 2: Low-FODMAP Quinoa Tabbouleh

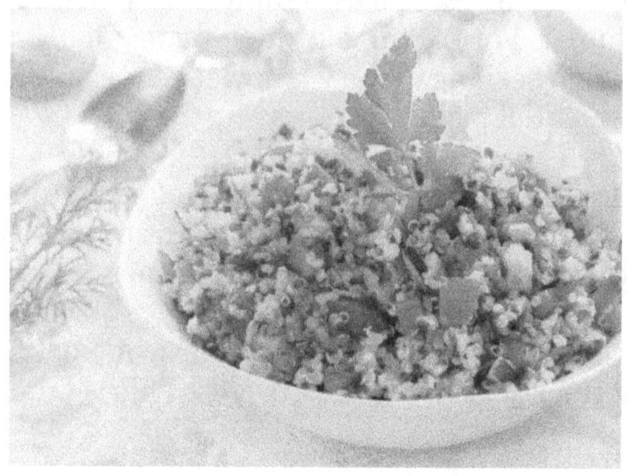

- **P. T. :** 30 minutes
- **Ingr. :** 1 cup of cooked quinoa, 1 cup of finely chopped flat-leaf parsley, 4 medium tomatoes, diced, 1 cucumber, diced, 2 tablespoons of garlic-infused olive oil, Juice of 1 lemon, Salt and pepper to taste.
- **Servings :** Serves 4
- **M. of C. :** Mixing
- **Process:** Mix cooked quinoa, parsley, diced tomatoes, and cucumber in a large bowl. In a separate bowl, whisk together the garlic-infused olive oil, lemon juice, salt, and pepper to make a dressing. Pour the dressing over the quinoa mixture and toss to combine.
- **N. V. :** Each serving contains approximately 200 calories, 6g of protein, 7g of fat, 28g of carbohydrates, and 5g of fiber.

Recipe 3: Low-FODMAP Greek Pasta Salad

- **P. T. :** 25 minutes
- **Ingr. :** 2 cups cooked gluten-free pasta, 1 cup diced cucumber, 1/2 cup sliced Kalamata olives, 1/2 cup crumbled feta cheese, 1/4 cup red wine vinegar, 2 tablespoons olive oil, 1 teaspoon dried oregano, salt and pepper to taste.
- **Servings :** Serves 4
- **M. of C. :** Mixing
- **Process:** In a large bowl, mix together the pasta, cucumber, olives, and feta. In a separate small bowl, whisk together the vinegar, oil, oregano, salt, and pepper to create a dressing. Drizzle the dressing over the pasta mixture and toss until well combined. Refrigerate until ready to serve.
- **N. V. :** Each serving contains approximately 320 calories, 8g of protein, 14g of fat, 40g of carbohydrates, and 3g of fiber.

Recipe 4: Low-FODMAP Baked Salmon with Dill

- **P. T. :** 30 minutes
- **Ingr. :** 2 salmon fillets, 2 tablespoons of lemon juice, 2 tablespoons of olive oil, 1 tablespoon of fresh dill, chopped, salt and pepper to taste.
- **Servings :** Serves 2

- **M. of C. :** Baking
- **Process:** Preheat the oven to 400°F (200°C). Place the salmon fillets on a baking sheet. Drizzle with lemon juice and olive oil, then sprinkle with dill, salt, and pepper. Bake for 15-20 minutes, or until the salmon is cooked through.
- **N. V. :** Each serving contains approximately 350 calories, 34g of protein, 23g of fat, 0g of carbohydrates, and 0g of fiber.

Recipe 5: Low-FODMAP Roasted Vegetable Frittata

- **P. T. :** 45 minutes
- **Ingr. :** 6 eggs, 1/4 cup of lactose-free milk, 2 cups of assorted roasted vegetables (like bell peppers, zucchini, and eggplant), 1/2 cup of crumbled feta cheese, salt and pepper to taste.
- **Servings :** Serves 4
- **M. of C. :** Baking
- **Process:** Preheat the oven to 375°F (190°C). In a large bowl, whisk together the eggs, milk, salt, and pepper. Stir in the roasted vegetables and feta. Pour the mixture into a greased pie dish. Bake for 25-30 minutes, or until the frittata is set.
- **N. V. :** Each serving contains approximately 200 calories, 13g of protein, 12g of fat, 10g of carbohydrates, and 3g of fiber.

Recipe 6: Low-FODMAP Chicken Stir-Fry

- **P. T. :** 30 minutes
- **Ingr. :** 2 skinless chicken breasts, cut into strips, 2 tablespoons of garlic-infused oil, 2 cups of mixed low-FODMAP vegetables (like bell peppers, carrots, and bok choy), 2 tablespoons of gluten-free soy sauce, 1 tablespoon of rice vinegar, 1 teaspoon of ginger paste.
- **Servings :** Serves 2
- **M. of C. :** Stir-frying
- **Process:** Heat the oil in a wok or large frying pan over medium-high heat. Add the chicken and cook until browned. Add the vegetables and stir-fry for a few more minutes. In a small bowl, combine the soy sauce, vinegar, and ginger. Pour the sauce over the chicken and vegetables, then stir well to combine.
- **N. V. :** Each serving contains approximately 340 calories, 30g of protein, 14g of fat, 20g of carbohydrates, and 4g of fiber.

Recipe 7: Low-FODMAP Beef Tacos

- **P. T. :** 20 minutes
- **Ingr. :** 1 lb lean ground beef, 1 tablespoon garlic-infused oil, 1 cup diced tomatoes, 1/2 cup chopped scallions (green parts only), 1 tablespoon taco seasoning, 8 corn tortillas, Optional toppings: shredded lettuce, diced tomatoes, cheddar cheese.
- **Servings :** Serves 4
- **M. of C. :** Sautéing
- **Process:** Heat the oil in a pan over medium-high heat. Add the ground beef and cook until browned, breaking it up into small pieces. Stir in the tomatoes, scallions, and taco seasoning. Cook for a few more minutes until well combined. Serve

the beef mixture on the corn tortillas with your choice of toppings.
- **N. V. :** Each serving (two tacos) contains approximately 340 calories, 24g of protein, 14g of fat, 26g of carbohydrates, and 4g of fiber.

Recipe 8: Low-FODMAP Vegetable Curry

- **P. T. :** 40 minutes
- **Ingr. :** 2 tablespoons coconut oil, 1 cup diced tomatoes, 1 cup diced eggplant, 1 cup diced zucchini, 1/2 cup diced red bell pepper, 1/4 cup chopped fresh cilantro, 2 tablespoons curry powder, 1 can coconut milk, Salt to taste.
- **Servings :** Serves 4
- **M. of C. :** Simmering
- **Process:** Heat the oil in a large pot over medium heat. Add the vegetables and cook until they start to soften. Stir in the curry powder until the vegetables are well coated. Add the coconut milk and simmer until the vegetables are tender and the flavors are well blended. Stir in the cilantro and salt to taste just before serving.
- **N. V. :** Each serving contains approximately 260 calories, 4g of protein, 20g of fat, 20g of carbohydrates, and 5g of fiber.

Recipe 9: Low-FODMAP Quinoa Salad

- **P. T. :** 30 minutes
- **Ingr. :** 1 cup cooked quinoa, 1 cup diced cucumber, 1 cup halved cherry tomatoes, 1/4 cup chopped scallions (green parts only), 2 tablespoons olive oil, 1 tablespoon lemon juice, Salt and pepper to taste.
- **Servings :** Serves 4
- **M. of C. :** Mixing
- **Process:** In a large bowl, combine the quinoa, cucumber, tomatoes, and scallions. In a small bowl, whisk together the olive oil, lemon juice, salt, and pepper to make a dressing. Pour the dressing over the quinoa mixture and toss until well combined.
- **N. V. :** Each serving contains approximately 180 calories, 4g of protein, 7g of fat, 25g of carbohydrates, and 3g of fiber.

Recipe 10: Low-FODMAP Grilled Shrimp Skewers

- **P. T. :** 25 minutes
- **Ingr. :** 1 lb large shrimp, peeled and deveined, 2 tablespoons olive oil, 1 tablespoon lemon juice, 1 tablespoon chopped fresh parsley, Salt and pepper to taste.
- **Servings :** Serves 4
- **M. of C. :** Grilling
- **Process:** Preheat a grill to medium-high heat. Toss the shrimp with the olive oil, lemon juice, parsley, salt, and pepper. Thread the shrimp onto skewers. Grill for 2-3 minutes per side, or until the shrimp are pink and cooked through.
- **N. V. :** Each serving contains approximately 170 calories, 24g of protein, 7g of fat, 0g of carbohydrates, and 0g of fiber.

Recipe 11: Low-FODMAP Chicken Stir-Fry

- **P. T. :** 25 minutes
- **Ingr. :** 1 lb boneless, skinless chicken breasts (cut into thin strips), 1 tablespoon garlic-infused oil, 1 cup diced bell pepper, 1/2 cup chopped scallions (green parts only), 2 tablespoons soy sauce (gluten-free, if needed), 1 tablespoon rice vinegar.
- **Servings :** Serves 4
- **M. of C. :** Stir-frying
- **Process:** Heat the oil in a wok or large frying pan over high heat. Add the chicken and cook until it's no longer pink. Add the bell pepper and scallions, and stir-fry for a couple more minutes. Stir in the soy sauce and rice vinegar and cook for another minute or two until everything is well combined and heated through.
- **N. V. :** Each serving contains approximately 220 calories, 30g of protein, 7g of fat, 6g of carbohydrates, and 1g of fiber.

Recipe 12: Low-FODMAP Spinach and Feta Frittata

- **P. T. :** 35 minutes
- **Ingr. :** 8 eggs, 1/2 cup lactose-free milk, 1 cup chopped fresh spinach, 1/2 cup crumbled feta cheese, Salt and pepper to taste.
- **Servings :** Serves 4
- **M. of C. :** Baking
- **Process:** Preheat your oven to 375 degrees Fahrenheit (190 degrees Celsius). In a large bowl, whisk together the eggs, milk, salt, and pepper. Stir in the spinach and feta. Pour the mixture into a greased pie dish and bake for 25-30 minutes, or until the eggs are set and the top is lightly browned.
- **N. V. :** Each serving contains approximately 220 calories, 18g of protein, 15g of fat, 3g of carbohydrates, and 1g of fiber.

Recipe 13: Low-FODMAP Stuffed Bell Peppers

- **P. T. :** 50 minutes
- **Ingr. :** 4 bell peppers, 1 lb lean ground beef, 1 cup cooked quinoa, 1 cup diced tomatoes, 1/2 cup chopped scallions (green parts only), Salt and pepper to taste.
- **Servings :** Serves 4
- **M. of C. :** Baking
- **Process:** Preheat your oven to 375 degrees Fahrenheit (190 degrees Celsius). Cut off the tops of the peppers and remove the seeds. In a large bowl, mix together the ground beef, quinoa, tomatoes, scallions, salt, and pepper. Stuff the mixture into the peppers and place them in a baking dish. Bake for 30-35 minutes, or until the peppers are tender and the filling is cooked through.
- **N. V. :** Each serving contains approximately 340 calories, 28g of protein, 12g of fat, 28g of carbohydrates, and 6g of fiber.

Recipe 14: Low-FODMAP Tuna Salad

- **P. T. :** 10 minutes
- **Ingr. :** 2 cans tuna (drained), 1/4 cup mayonnaise (lactose-free, if needed), 1/4 cup diced celery, 1/4 cup chopped scallions (green parts only), Salt and pepper to taste.
- **Servings :** Serves 4
- **M. of C. :** Mixing
- **Process:** In a large bowl, mix together the tuna, mayonnaise, celery, and scallions. Season with salt and

pepper to taste. Serve on a bed of lettuce or as a sandwich filling.

- **N. V. :** Each serving contains approximately 190 calories, 20g of protein, 10g of fat, 1g of carbohydrates, and 0g of fiber.

Recipe 15: Low-FODMAP Shrimp Scampi

- **P. T. :** 20 minutes
- **Ingr. :** 1 lb large shrimp (peeled and deveined), 2 tablespoons garlic-infused oil, 1/2 cup white wine, 1/2 cup chopped fresh parsley, Salt and pepper to taste.
- **Servings :** Serves 4
- **M. of C. :** Sautéing
- **Process:** Heat the oil in a large pan over medium heat. Add the shrimp and cook until they turn pink. Remove the shrimp from the pan. Add the wine to the pan and simmer for a couple of minutes. Return the shrimp to the pan, stir in the parsley, and season with salt and pepper. Cook for another minute or two until everything is heated through.
- **N. V. :** Each serving contains approximately 230 calories, 24g of protein, 10g of fat, 2g of carbohydrates, and 0g of fiber.

Recipe 16: Low-FODMAP Greek Salad

- **P. T. :** 15 minutes
- **Ingr. :** 4 cups chopped romaine lettuce, 1 cup diced cucumber, 1/2 cup diced tomatoes, 1/2 cup sliced kalamata olives, 1/2 cup crumbled feta cheese, 1/4 cup olive oil, 2 tablespoons red wine vinegar, Salt and pepper to taste.
- **Servings :** Serves 4
- **M. of C. :** Mixing
- **Process:** In a large bowl, combine the lettuce, cucumber, tomatoes, olives, and feta. In a small bowl, whisk together the olive oil, vinegar, salt, and pepper. Drizzle the dressing over the salad and toss to combine.
- **N. V. :** Each serving contains approximately 250 calories, 6g of protein, 20g of fat, 8g of carbohydrates, and 3g of fiber.

Recipe 17: Low-FODMAP Quinoa Salad

- **P. T. :** 30 minutes
- **Ingr. :** 1 cup quinoa, 2 cups water, 1 cup diced cucumber, 1/2 cup diced tomatoes, 1/2 cup chopped scallions (green parts only), 1/4 cup olive oil, 2 tablespoons lemon juice, Salt and pepper to taste.
- **Servings :** Serves 4
- **M. of C. :** Boiling, Mixing
- **Process:** In a saucepan, bring the quinoa and water to a boil. Reduce the heat to low, cover the pan, and simmer for 15-20 minutes until the quinoa is tender and the water is absorbed. Let the quinoa cool. In a large bowl, combine the cooled quinoa, cucumber, tomatoes, and scallions. In a small bowl, whisk together the olive oil, lemon juice, salt, and pepper. Drizzle the dressing over the salad and toss to combine.
- **N. V. :** Each serving contains approximately 260 calories, 6g of protein, 14g of fat, 28g of carbohydrates, and 3g of fiber.

Recipe 18: Low-FODMAP Turkey Wraps

- **P. T. :** 10 minutes
- **Ingr. :** 4 gluten-free tortillas, 1/2 lb sliced turkey, 1/4 cup mayonnaise (lactose-free, if needed), 1 cup lettuce, 1/2 cup diced tomatoes.
- **Servings :** Serves 4
- **M. of C. :** Assembling
- **Process:** Spread each tortilla with a tablespoon of mayonnaise. Layer the turkey, lettuce, and tomatoes on top of the tortillas. Roll up the tortillas and slice them in half.
- **N. V. :** Each serving contains approximately 240 calories, 14g of protein, 10g of fat, 26g of carbohydrates, and 3g of fiber.

Recipe 19: Low-FODMAP Grilled Chicken with Zucchini

- **P. T. :** 25 minutes
- **Ingr. :** 2 boneless, skinless chicken breasts, 2 medium-sized zucchinis (cut into rounds), 2 tablespoons garlic-infused oil, Salt and pepper to taste.
- **Servings :** Serves 2
- **M. of C. :** Grilling
- **Process:** Preheat your grill on medium heat. Brush the chicken breasts and zucchini rounds with garlic-infused oil and season with salt and pepper. Place the chicken and zucchini on the grill and cook for 6-8 minutes on each side, or until the chicken is cooked through and the zucchini is tender.
- **N. V. :** Each serving contains approximately 290 calories, 30g of protein, 13g of fat, 10g of carbohydrates, and 3g of fiber.

Recipe 20: Low-FODMAP Vegetable Stir Fry

- **P. T. :** 20 minutes
- **Ingr. :** 2 tablespoons garlic-infused oil, 2 medium-sized carrots (sliced into rounds), 1 red bell pepper (diced), 1 zucchini (diced), 2 tablespoons low-sodium soy sauce, Salt and pepper to taste.
- **Servings :** Serves 2
- **M. of C. :** Stir-Frying
- **Process:** Heat the oil in a large pan over medium-high heat. Add the carrots, bell pepper, and zucchini and stir-fry for 5-7 minutes until the vegetables are tender-crisp. Add the soy sauce and season with salt and pepper. Stir to combine and cook for another minute or two until everything is heated through.
- **N.V. :** Each serving contains approximately 170 calories, 3g of protein, 14g of fat, 12g of carbohydrates, and 3g of fiber.

With these recipes, you now have a diverse and delicious selection of low-FODMAP lunch recipes at your disposal. Remember that a balanced and varied diet is key to managing your IBS symptoms effectively. Enjoy your lunch!

Chapter 5: Dinner Recipes

Introduction to Dinner

Dinner, often considered the day's grand finale, is not just about satisfying hunger—it's a harmonious blend of comfort and nourishment, the perfect closure to the day. While cultural norms may influence what dinner looks like globally, we focus on the potential of creating delightful, delicious, and digestive-friendly meals following a low-FODMAP diet.

Many believe that following a low-FODMAP diet restricts your dinner options, but that's far from the truth. This chapter aims to debunk that myth and showcase a wide array of tantalizing, gut-friendly dinners that align with a low-FODMAP lifestyle.

The upcoming recipes balance simplicity and creativity, catering to varied tastes and schedules. Whether you're looking for a quick weekday meal or a more elaborate weekend dinner, you'll find recipes that celebrate the union of flavor and gut-friendly nutrition. These meals demonstrate that a satisfying, flavorful dinner can coexist beautifully with a low-FODMAP lifestyle.

So let's embark on this culinary adventure together, savoring low-FODMAP dinners that bring joy to your tastebuds and wellness to your gut.

Dinner Recipes

Recipe 1: Hearty Ratatouille

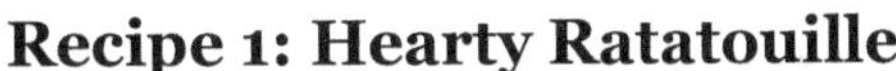

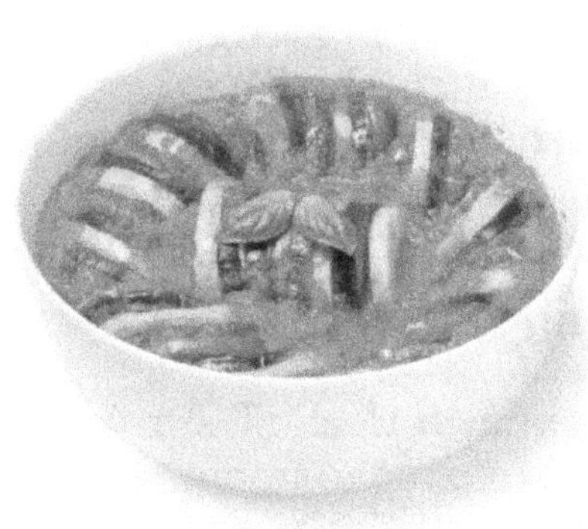

- **Ingr. :** Eggplant, zucchinis, bell peppers, tomatoes, onions, garlic, olive oil, herbes de Provence.
- **Serv. :** 6
- **M. of C. :** Roasting
- **Process:** Dice all the vegetables into bite-size pieces. Heat oil in a large pot, add onions and garlic until translucent. Add other vegetables, cover, and cook for 40 minutes, stirring occasionally.
- **N. V. (for serving):** Calories: 150, Protein: 3.8g, Fat: 7.2g, Carbohydrates: 20.4g, Fiber: 7g

- **P. T. :** 15 minutes
- **C. T. :** 45 minutes

Recipe 2: Quinoa-Stuffed Bell Peppers

- **P. T. :** 20 minutes
- **C. T. :** 30 minutes
- **Ingr. :** Quinoa, bell peppers, black beans, corn, diced tomatoes, spices.
- **Serv. :** 4
- **M. of C. :** Baking
- **Process:** Cook quinoa as per instructions. Cut the tops off bell peppers, remove the insides. Mix quinoa with beans, corn, tomatoes, and spices. Stuff the peppers and bake for 30 minutes.
- **N. V. (for serving):** Calories: 265, Protein: 10.2g, Fat: 5.8g, Carbohydrates: 45.3g, Fiber: 8.9g

Recipe 3: Maple Glazed Salmon

- **P. T. :** 10 minutes
- **C. T. :** 15 minutes
- **Ingr. :** Salmon fillets, maple syrup, soy sauce, garlic, black pepper.
- **Serv. :** 4
- **M. of C. :** Baking
- **Process:** Mix maple syrup, soy sauce, garlic, and black pepper. Marinade salmon for 10 minutes. Bake for 15 minutes or until cooked through.
- **N. V. (for serving):** Calories: 265, Protein: 22.1g, Fat: 13.2g, Carbohydrates: 16.8g, Fiber: 0g

Recipe 4: Lemon Herb Chicken

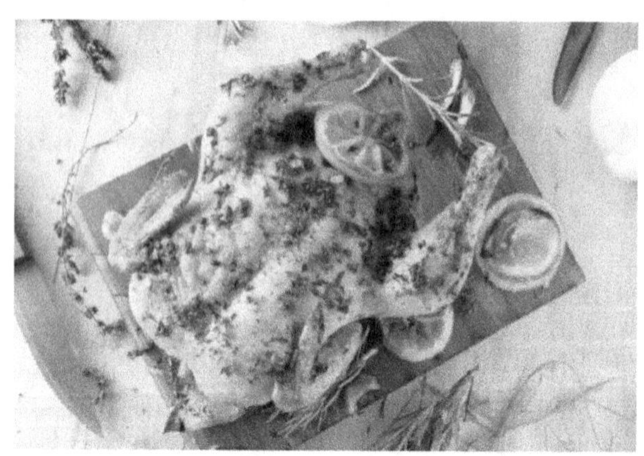

- **P. T. :** 15 minutes
- **C. T. :** 25 minutes
- **Ingr. :** Chicken breasts, lemon juice, mixed herbs, olive oil, salt, pepper.
- **Serv. :** 4
- **M. of C. :** Grilling
- **Process:** Mix lemon juice, herbs, oil, salt, and pepper. Marinade chicken for 10 minutes. Grill on medium heat until cooked through.
- **N. V. (for serving):** Calories: 287, Protein: 30.8g, Fat: 16.2g, Carbohydrates: 2.6g, Fiber: 0.8g

Recipe 5: Low-FODMAP Vegetable Stir-fry

- **P. T. :** 15 minutes
- **C. T. :** 20 minutes
- **Ingr. :** Carrots, bell peppers, zucchini, tofu, sesame oil, gluten-free soy sauce, ginger.
- **Serv. :** 4
- **M. of C. :** Stir-frying
- **Process:** Heat oil, stir-fry veggies, and tofu for 10 minutes. Add soy sauce and ginger, stir-fry for another 10 minutes.
- **N. V. (for serving):** Calories: 217, Protein: 10.5g, Fat: 15.2g, Carbohydrates: 14.8g, Fiber: 3.2g

Recipe 6: Quinoa Stuffed Bell Peppers

- **P. T. :** 15 minutes
- **C. T. :** 25 minutes
- **Ingr. :** Quinoa, bell peppers, tomatoes, onions, cumin, olive oil, salt, pepper.
- **Serv. :** 4
- **M. of C. :** Baking

- **Process:** Cook quinoa, mix with chopped tomatoes and onions, season with cumin, salt, and pepper. Stuff bell peppers with the mixture, drizzle oil, and bake for 25 minutes.
- **N. V. (for serving):** Calories: 243, Protein: 8.1g, Fat: 10.2g, Carbohydrates: 32.6g, Fiber: 5.9g

Recipe 7: Lemon Herb Baked Cod

- **P. T. :** 10 minutes
- **C. T. :** 15 minutes
- **Ingr. :** Cod fillets, lemon juice, fresh herbs (parsley, dill), olive oil, salt, pepper.
- **Serv. :** 4
- **M. of C. :** Baking

- **Process:** Marinate the cod in lemon juice, herbs, oil, salt, and pepper. Bake for 15 minutes or until flaky.
- **N. V. (for serving):** Calories: 189, Protein: 22.1g, Fat: 9.7g, Carbohydrates: 2.2g, Fiber: 0.3g

Recipe 8: Low-FODMAP Beef Stir-fry

- **P. T. :** 15 minutes
- **C. T. :** 20 minutes
- **Ingr. :** Beef strips, bell peppers, carrots, bok choy, garlic-infused oil, gluten-free soy sauce.
- **Serv. :** 4
- **M. of C. :** Stir-frying

- **Process:** Heat oil, stir-fry beef until browned, add veggies, and stir-fry for another 10 minutes. Add soy sauce, stir well, and serve.
- **N. V. (for serving):** Calories: 283, Protein: 25.8g, Fat: 15.3g, Carbohydrates: 10.5g, Fiber: 2.7g

Recipe 9: Chicken Quinoa Salad

- **P. T. :** 20 minutes
- **C. T. :** 30 minutes
- **Ingr. :** Quinoa, chicken breast, cherry tomatoes, cucumber, feta cheese, olives, lemon juice, olive oil, salt, pepper.
- **Serv. :** 4
- **M. of C. :** Boiling, Grilling

- **Process:** Cook quinoa as per instructions. Grill chicken until done. Chop veggies, mix everything, and season.
- **N. V. (for serving):** Calories: 310, Protein: 28g, Fat: 12g, Carbohydrates: 23g, Fiber: 3g

Recipe 10: Shrimp Pasta with Zucchini

- **P. T. :** 15 minutes
- **C. T. :** 15 minutes

- **Ingr. :** Gluten-free pasta, shrimp, zucchini, garlic-infused oil, lemon zest, chili flakes, parsley, salt.
- **Serv. :** 4

- **M. of C. :** Boiling, Sautéing
- **Process:** Cook pasta, sauté shrimp and zucchini in oil. Mix with pasta, add lemon zest, chili, parsley, and salt.
- **N. V. (for serving):** Calories: 365, Protein: 25g, Fat: 8g, Carbohydrates: 50g, Fiber: 3g

Recipe 11: Baked Salmon with Dill Sauce

- **P. T. :** 10 minutes
- **C. T. :** 20 minutes
- **Ingr. :** Salmon fillets, olive oil, salt, pepper, fresh dill, lemon juice, garlic-infused oil, Dijon mustard.
- **Serv. :** 4
- **M. of C. :** Baking
- **Process:** Season and bake salmon. Mix dill, lemon juice, oil, and mustard for sauce. Serve salmon with sauce.
- **N. V. (for serving):** Calories: 345, Protein: 34g, Fat: 21g, Carbohydrates: 2g, Fiber: 0g

Recipe 12: Beef Stir-Fry with Bell Peppers

- **P. T. :** 15 minutes
- **C. T. :** 10 minutes
- **Ingr. :** Beef sirloin, bell peppers, garlic-infused oil, ginger, low-sodium soy sauce, scallions.
- **Serv. :** 4
- **M. of C. :** Stir-frying
- **Process:** Stir-fry beef, remove. Stir-fry peppers, ginger, add beef, soy sauce. Garnish with scallions.
- **N. V. (for serving):** Calories: 335, Protein: 25g, Fat: 22g, Carbohydrates: 8g, Fiber: 2g

Recipe 13: Low-FODMAP Chicken Caesar Salad

- **P. T. :** 15 minutes
- **C. T. :** 15 minutes
- **Ingr. :** Chicken breasts, Romaine lettuce, Parmesan cheese, gluten-free croutons, garlic-infused oil, lemon juice, Dijon mustard, egg yolk.
- **Serv. :** 4
- **M. of C. :** Grilling, tossing
- **Process:** Grill chicken. Prepare salad dressing with oil, lemon juice, mustard, yolk. Toss lettuce, cheese, croutons, dressing. Top with sliced chicken.
- **N. V. (for serving):** Calories: 325, Protein: 28g, Fat: 20g, Carbohydrates: 7g, Fiber: 2g

Recipe 14: Vegetable Lasagna with Spinach and Zucchini

- **P. T. :** 30 minutes
- **C. T. :** 45 minutes
- **Ingr. :** Gluten-free lasagna noodles, spinach, zucchini, ricotta cheese, mozzarella cheese, low-FODMAP marinara sauce.
- **Serv. :** 6
- **M. of C. :** Baking
- **Process:** Cook noodles. Layer noodles, spinach, zucchini, cheeses, sauce in a baking dish. Bake until bubbly and golden.
- **N. V. (for serving):** Calories: 460, Protein: 20g, Fat: 21g, Carbohydrates: 50g, Fiber: 3g

Recipe 15: Low-FODMAP Pad Thai

- **P. T. :** 15 minutes
- **C. T. :** 20 minutes
- **Ingr. :** Rice noodles, shrimp, bell peppers, carrot, egg, green onion tops, peanut oil, gluten-free soy sauce, lime, sugar, crushed peanuts.
- **Serv. :** 4
- **M. of C. :** Stir-frying
- **Process:** Cook noodles. Stir-fry shrimp, vegetables, egg in oil. Mix in cooked noodles, soy sauce, lime juice, sugar. Garnish with peanuts.
- **N. V. (for serving):** Calories: 410, Protein: 20g, Fat: 15g, Carbohydrates: 55g, Fiber: 3g

Recipe 16: Grilled Salmon with Dill Sauce

- **P. T. :** 10 minutes
- **C. T. :** 15 minutes
- **Ingr. :** Salmon fillets, lemon juice, olive oil, dill, low-FODMAP mayonnaise, Dijon mustard, green onion tops.
- **Serv. :** 4
- **M. of C. :** Grilling
- **Process:** Grill salmon. Prepare sauce with mayonnaise, dill, mustard, green onion tops. Serve salmon with sauce.
- **N. V. (for serving):** Calories: 405, Protein: 34g, Fat: 28g, Carbohydrates: 2g, Fiber: 0g

Recipe 17: Baked Lemon Herb Chicken

- **P. T. :** 15 minutes
- **C. T. :** 25 minutes
- **Ingr. :** Chicken breasts, lemon juice, olive oil, garlic-infused oil, fresh thyme, fresh rosemary, salt, pepper.
- **Serv. :** 4
- **M. of C. :** Baking
- **Process:** Marinate chicken in a mix of oils, lemon juice, herbs, salt, and pepper. Bake until golden and cooked through.
- **N. V. (for serving):** Calories: 275, Protein: 31g, Fat: 14g, Carbohydrates: 3g, Fiber: 0g

Recipe 18: Quinoa Salad with Veggies

- **P. T. :** 20 minutes
- **C. T. :** 15 minutes
- **Ingr. :** Quinoa, bell peppers, cucumber, cherry tomatoes, feta cheese, olive oil, lemon juice, salt, pepper. lemon juice. Season with salt and pepper.
- **M. of C. :** Boiling and Tossing
- **Process:** Cook quinoa. Toss quinoa with diced vegetables, crumbled feta cheese, and a dressing of olive oil and
- **Serv. :** 4
- **N. V. (for serving):** Calories: 310, Protein: 11g, Fat: 12g, Carbohydrates: 41g, Fiber: 6g

Recipe 19: Grilled Vegetable Skewers

- **P. T. :** 20 minutes
- **C. T. :** 10 minutes
- **Ingr. :** Zucchini, bell peppers, cherry tomatoes, red onion, garlic-infused oil, salt, pepper.
- **Serv. :** 4

- **M. of C. :** Grilling
- **Process:** Skewer cut veggies and brush with garlic-infused oil, salt, and pepper. Grill until veggies are tender and slightly charred.
- **N. V. (for serving):** Calories: 100, Protein: 3g, Fat: 4g, Carbohydrates: 15g, Fiber: 4g

Recipe 20: Shrimp Stir-fry with Buckwheat Noodles

- **P. T. :** 15 minutes
- **C. T. :** 20 minutes
- **Ingr. :** Shrimp, buckwheat noodles, bell peppers, carrots, sesame oil, low sodium soy sauce, ginger, garlic-infused oil, green onions.
- **Serv. :** 4
- **M. of C. :** Stir-frying
- **Process:** Stir-fry shrimp and veggies in a mix of oils, ginger, and soy sauce. Toss with cooked buckwheat noodles and top with green onions.
- **N. V. (for serving):** Calories: 365, Protein: 25g, Fat: 10g, Carbohydrates: 45g, Fiber: 5g

And there you have it! Twenty delicious, diverse, and low-FODMAP dinner recipes. Each one crafted with love and consideration for those managing IBS symptoms, seeking a healthier lifestyle, or simply looking to diversify their dinner menu. So go ahead, give them a try and enjoy a culinary journey like no other. Bon appétit!

Chapter 6: Snacks and Appetizers

Introduction to Snacks and Appetizers

In this chapter, we dive into the vibrant world of low-FODMAP snacks and appetizers. Snacks are not just hunger-busters, they're integral to our daily nutrition. Appetizers, the opening act of any meal, set the tone for what's to follow.

For those following a low-FODMAP diet, finding suitable snacks and appetizers may feel daunting. This chapter aims to change that, featuring a variety of recipes that make snacking enjoyable and digestion-friendly.

Creating delicious, crowd-pleasing snacks and appetizers that remain low-FODMAP is achievable with the right recipes and ingredients. Whether you're in need of a quick bite or a sophisticated starter for a dinner party, we've got you covered.

Embracing a low-FODMAP diet is about exploring new flavors and combinations that satisfy your taste buds while being kind to your gut. Welcome to the exciting world of low-FODMAP snacks and appetizers where flavor meets health and every bite brings you closer to better wellbeing. Let's transform snacking and appetizing into a delicious, stress-free part of your life.

Detailed recipes

Recipe 1: Zesty Lentil Hummus

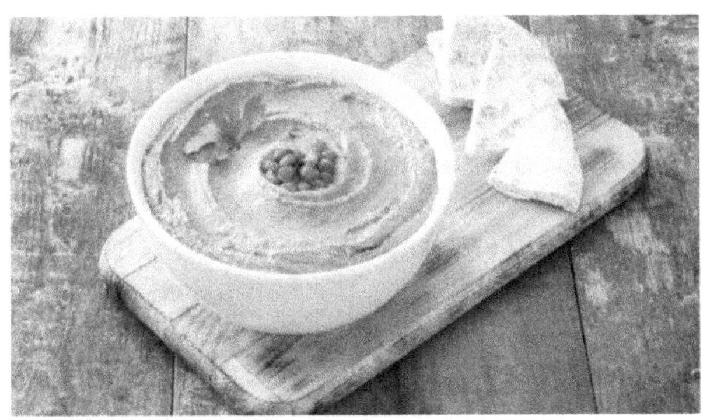

- **P. T. :** 15 minutes
- **Ingr. :** 2 cups of cooked lentils, 2 cloves of garlic, juice of 2 lemons, 2 tbsp of tahini, salt to taste, 2 tbsp of olive oil, paprika for garnish.
- Servings : Serves 4
- **M. of C. :** Blending
- **Process:** Combine the cooked lentils, garlic, lemon juice, tahini, and salt in a blender. Blend until smooth. Slowly drizzle in the olive oil while the blender is running. Garnish with paprika before serving.
- **N. V. :** Per serving: 183 calories, 8g protein, 25g carbohydrates, 6g fat, 7g fiber.

Recipe 2: Quinoa and Black Bean Salad

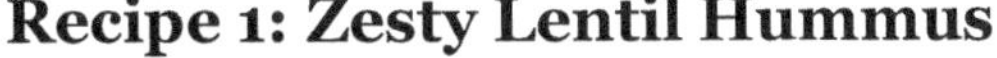

- **P. T. :** 30 minutes
- **Ingr. :** 1 cup of quinoa, 2 cups of water, 1 can of black beans, 1 red bell pepper, 1 green bell pepper, 1 red onion, 1/2 cup of cilantro, 1/4 cup of lime juice, 2 tbsp of olive oil, salt and pepper to taste.
- Servings : Serves 6
- **M. of C. :** Boiling, Mixing
- **Process:** Cook quinoa in boiling water according to package instructions. Drain and rinse black beans. Dice bell peppers and onion, chop cilantro. Combine all ingredients in a large bowl and mix well.
- **N. V. :** Per serving: 220 calories, 8g protein, 37g carbohydrates, 6g fat, 8g fiber.

Recipe 3: Crunchy Kale Chips

- **P. T. :** 30 minutes
- **Ingr. :** 1 bunch of kale, 1 tablespoon of olive oil, 1/2 teaspoon of sea salt.
- Servings : Serves 2
- **M. of C. :** Baking
- **Process:** Preheat the oven to 300 degrees F (150 degrees C). Remove the kale leaves from the thick stems and tear into bite-sized pieces. Toss with olive oil and salt. Bake for 10-15 minutes until crisp but not browned.
- **N. V. :** Per serving: 93 calories, 2.2g protein, 7.4g carbohydrates, 7.1g fat, 1.3g fiber.

Recipe 4: Sweet Potato and Avocado Bites

- **P. T. :** 20 minutes
- **Ingr. :** 2 sweet potatoes, 1 avocado, juice of 1 lime, 1/4 cup of chopped cilantro, salt to taste.
- Servings : Serves 4
- **M. of C. :** Baking, Mixing
- **Process:** Preheat oven to 400 degrees F (200 degrees C). Slice the sweet potatoes into 1/4 inch rounds and bake for 10 minutes on each side. In the meantime, mash the avocado and mix with lime juice, cilantro, and salt. Once the sweet potatoes are done, top each slice with the avocado mixture.
- **N. V. :** Per serving: 145 calories, 2.2g protein, 18g carbohydrates, 7.8g fat, 5g fiber.

Recipe 5: Tangy Tuna Stuffed Tomatoes

- **P. T. :** 15 minutes
- **Ingr. :** 4 medium tomatoes, 2 cans of tuna, 1/4 cup of low-fat mayo, 1/2 cup of chopped celery, salt and pepper to taste.
- Servings : Serves 4
- **M. of C. :** Mixing
- **Process:** Slice the tops of the tomatoes and hollow out the insides. In a bowl, mix the tuna, mayo, celery, and seasoning. Spoon the tuna mixture into the tomatoes.
- **N. V. :** Per serving: 158 calories, 22.1g protein, 8g carbohydrates, 4.6g fat, 1.8g fiber.

Recipe 6: Spicy Edamame Dip

- **P. T. :** 15 minutes
- **Ingr. :** 2 cups of shelled edamame, 1/4 cup of tahini, 1/4 cup of water, 1/2 teaspoon of crushed red pepper flakes, 2 cloves of garlic, juice of 1 lemon, salt to taste.
- Servings : Serves 4
- **M. of C. :** Blending

- **Process:** In a food processor, combine all the ingredients and blend until smooth. Adjust seasoning to taste.

- **N. V. :** Per serving: 197 calories, 12.4g protein, 14.1g carbohydrates, 10.4g fat, 5.1g fiber.

Recipe 7: Lemon Herb Chicken Skewers

- **P. T. :** 25 minutes + 2 hours for marination
- **Ingr. :** 500g chicken breast, 2 lemons, 3 cloves garlic, a handful of fresh parsley, 2 tbsp olive oil, salt and pepper to taste.
- Servings : Serves 4
- **M. of C. :** Grilling
- **Process:** Cut the chicken into bite-sized pieces. In a bowl, combine the juice of the lemons, minced garlic, chopped parsley, olive oil, salt, and pepper. Marinate the chicken in this mixture for at least 2 hours. Thread the chicken onto skewers and grill until cooked through.
- **N. V. :** Per serving: 230 calories, 30g protein, 3g carbohydrates, 11g fat, 0g fiber.

Recipe 8: Vegan Carrot Hummus

- **P. T. :** 10 minutes
- **Ingr. :** 2 cups cooked carrots, 1 cup chickpeas, 2 cloves garlic, 2 tbsp tahini, juice of 1 lemon, salt to taste.
- Servings : Serves 4
- **M. of C. :** Blending
- **Process:** Blend all the ingredients together in a food processor until smooth. Adjust seasoning to taste.
- **N. V. :** Per serving: 130 calories, 5g protein, 20g carbohydrates, 4g fat, 5g fiber.

Recipe 9: Spiced Roasted Chickpeas

- **P. T. :** 45 minutes
- **Ingr. :** 2 cups chickpeas, 1 tbsp olive oil, 1 tsp paprika, 1/2 tsp turmeric, salt and pepper to taste.
- Servings : Serves 4
- **M. of C. :** Baking
- **Process:** Preheat your oven to 200°C (390°F). Toss the chickpeas in olive oil and spices, then spread out on a baking sheet. Bake until crispy, about 30-40 minutes.
- **N. V. :** Per serving: 175 calories, 9g protein, 30g carbohydrates, 5g fat, 8g fiber.

Recipe 10: Watermelon and Feta Skewers

- **P. T. :** 10 minutes
- **Ingr. :** 2 cups watermelon cubes, 200g feta cheese, a handful of fresh mint leaves.
- Servings : Serves 4
- **M. of C. :** Assembling
- **Process:** Thread a piece of watermelon, a mint leaf, and a cube of feta onto a skewer. Repeat until all the ingredients are used.
- **N. V. :** Per serving: 130 calories, 5g protein, 15g carbohydrates, 6g fat, 1g fiber.

Recipe 11: Grilled Zucchini Rolls

- **P. T. :** 25 minutes
- **Ingr. :** 2 zucchinis, 1/2 cup ricotta cheese, 1/4 cup sun-dried tomatoes, 1/4 cup basil leaves.
- Servings : Serves 4
- **M. of C. :** Grilling
- **Process:** Cut the zucchinis into thin strips and grill for about 2 minutes on each side. Mix the ricotta cheese with sun-dried tomatoes. Roll a spoonful of the mixture in each zucchini strip and secure with a toothpick.
- **N. V. :** Per serving: 80 calories, 4g protein, 7g carbohydrates, 4g fat, 2g fiber.

Recipe 12: Sweet Potato Hummus

- **P. T. :** 40 minutes
- **Ingr. :** 2 medium sweet potatoes, 1 can of chickpeas, 2 tablespoons tahini, 2 garlic cloves, juice of 1 lemon, salt and pepper to taste.
- Servings : Serves 6
- **M. of C. :** Blending
- **Process:** Roast the sweet potatoes in the oven until soft. Combine the flesh of the sweet potatoes with the rest of the ingredients in a blender or food processor and blend until smooth.
- **N. V. :** Per serving: 160 calories, 5g protein, 25g carbohydrates, 5g fat, 6g fiber.

Recipe 13: Baked Veggie Spring Rolls

- **P. T. :** 50 minutes
- **Ingr. :** 12 rice paper wrappers, 1 cup shredded carrots, 1 cup shredded cabbage, 1 cup bean sprouts, 1 bell pepper thinly sliced, 1 tablespoon soy sauce, 1 teaspoon sesame oil.
- Servings : Serves 4
- **M. of C. :** Baking
- **Process:** Preheat the oven to 375°F (190°C). Combine the veggies, soy sauce, and sesame oil in a bowl. Soak the rice paper wrappers in warm water until they soften. Place a spoonful of the veggie mixture on each wrapper, roll them up, and bake for 20 minutes or until golden brown.
- **N. V. :** Per serving: 200 calories, 5g protein, 40g carbohydrates, 2g fat, 5g fiber.

Recipe 14: Greek Yogurt Parfait

- **P. T. :** 5 minutes
- **Ingr. :** 1 cup Greek yogurt, 1 tablespoon honey, 1/4 cup granola, 1/2 cup mixed berries.
- Servings : Serves 1
- **M. of C. :** No-cook
- **Process:** Layer Greek yogurt, honey, granola, and mixed berries in a glass or jar, repeating until all ingredients are used.
- **N. V. :** Per serving: 260 calories, 20g protein, 35g carbohydrates, 4g fat, 5g fiber.

Recipe 15: Zesty Quinoa Salad

- **P. T. :** 25 minutes

- **Ingr. :** 1 cup quinoa, 2 cups water, 1/4 cup extra-virgin olive oil, 2 limes, juiced, 2 teaspoons ground cumin, 1 teaspoon salt, 1/2 teaspoon red pepper flakes (optional), 1 1/2 cups halved cherry tomatoes, 1 (15 ounce) can black beans, drained and rinsed, 5 green onions, finely chopped, 1/4 cup chopped fresh cilantro.
- Servings : Serves 4
- **M. of C. :** Stovetop
- **Process:** Cook the quinoa according to package instructions. While the quinoa cools, combine olive oil, lime juice, cumin, salt, and red pepper flakes in a small bowl. Stir in tomatoes, black beans, and green onions into cooled quinoa. Pour dressing over quinoa mixture; toss to coat. Stir in cilantro; serve immediately or chill before serving.
- **N. V. :** Per serving: 430 calories, 15g protein, 60g carbohydrates, 15g fat, 13g fiber.

Recipe 16: Chickpea Hummus

- **P. T. :** 10 minutes
- **Ingr. :** 1 can chickpeas (drained and rinsed), 1 clove garlic, 2 tablespoons olive oil, 2 tablespoons tahini, Juice of 1 lemon, Salt to taste, Paprika for garnish (optional).
- Servings : Serves 4
- **M. of C. :** No-cook
- **Process:** Combine chickpeas, garlic, olive oil, tahini, lemon juice, and salt in a food processor or high-speed blender. Blend until smooth and creamy. If desired, garnish with a sprinkle of paprika.
- **N. V. :** Per serving: 210 calories, 7g protein, 20g carbohydrates, 12g fat, 6g fiber.

Recipe 17: Baked Sweet Potato Fries

- **P. T. :** 45 minutes
- **Ingr. :** 2 large sweet potatoes, 2 tablespoons olive oil, 1/2 teaspoon sea salt, 1/2 teaspoon paprika.
- Servings : Serves 4
- **M. of C. :** Baking
- **Process:** Preheat the oven to 200 degrees Celsius (400 degrees Fahrenheit). Cut the sweet potatoes into long, thin strips. Toss the sweet potato strips in a large bowl with olive oil, salt, and paprika. Arrange on a baking sheet in a single layer. Bake for 30 minutes or until crispy, turning once halfway through.
- **N. V. :** Per serving: 160 calories, 2g protein, 28g carbohydrates, 7g fat, 4g fiber.

Recipe 18: Vegan Stuffed Mushrooms

- **P. T. :** 30 minutes
- **Ingr. :** 12 large button mushrooms, 1 tablespoon olive oil, 1 onion (finely chopped), 2 cloves garlic (minced), 1 bell pepper (diced), 1/2 cup breadcrumbs, 1/2 cup vegan cheese, Salt and pepper to taste.
- Servings : Serves 4
- **M. of C. :** Baking
- **Process:** Preheat the oven to 200 degrees Celsius (400 degrees Fahrenheit). Remove stems from mushrooms and chop them finely. Heat olive oil in a pan, sauté onion, garlic, bell pepper, and chopped mushroom stems until soft. Stir in

breadcrumbs and vegan cheese, season with salt and pepper. Fill each mushroom cap with the mixture and place on a baking sheet. Bake for 15 minutes or until the mushrooms are soft and the filling is golden.

- **N. V. :** Per serving: 140 calories, 4g protein, 18g carbohydrates, 6g fat, 3g fiber

Recipe 19: Sesame Seed Encrusted Tofu Sticks

- **P. T. :** 35 minutes
- **Ingr. :** 1 pack of firm tofu, 1/2 cup sesame seeds, 2 tablespoons olive oil, 2 tablespoons soy sauce, 1 tablespoon maple syrup.
- Servings : Serves 4
- **M. of C. :** Baking
- **Process:** Preheat the oven to 180 degrees Celsius (350 degrees Fahrenheit). Drain the tofu and cut it into sticks. Mix the sesame seeds, olive oil, soy sauce, and maple syrup in a bowl. Coat each tofu stick in the sesame seed mixture and place them on a baking sheet. Bake for 20 minutes or until the tofu is golden and crispy.
- **N. V. :** Per serving: 220 calories, 15g protein, 10g carbohydrates, 15g fat, 3g fiber.

Recipe 20: Spicy Roasted Chickpeas

- **P. T. :** 45 minutes
- **Ingr. :** 2 cans of chickpeas, 2 tablespoons olive oil, 1 teaspoon chili powder, 1/2 teaspoon sea salt.
- Servings : Serves 6
- **M. of C. :** Roasting
- **Process:** Preheat the oven to 200 degrees Celsius (400 degrees Fahrenheit). Rinse and drain the chickpeas, pat them dry. In a large bowl, toss the chickpeas with olive oil, chili powder, and sea salt. Spread them out on a baking sheet and roast for 30 minutes or until crispy, stirring occasionally.
- **N. V. :** Per serving: 150 calories, 6g protein, 20g carbohydrates, 6g fat, 6g fiber.

These delightful snacks and appetizers are both satisfying and nutritious, perfect for those who want to manage their dietary requirements without compromising on flavor. Enjoy these treats and remember, the journey of exploration of various diets continues!

Chapter 7: Dessert

Introduction to Desserts

Delve into the captivating realm of Desserts, where guilty pleasures are transformed into wholesome delights. The recipes within this chapter have been meticulously curated to align with various nutritional needs, including managing IBS symptoms or maintaining fitness levels. We'll redefine desserts, proving they can be health-beneficial and satisfy your sweet cravings. This journey takes us beyond traditional desserts, emphasizing those that are as healthy as they are delicious. Through exploration of unconventional ingredients and substitutes, we broaden culinary horizons, enhancing your repertoire whether you're a novice cook or an experienced culinary artist.

Each dessert recipe includes preparation time, cooking time, serving size, required ingredients, detailed instructions, and nutritional values. This ensures a comprehensive understanding of creating various healthy desserts, enabling you to indulge in life's sweeter aspects without worry. Welcome to the wholesome world of delectable desserts. Let's embark on this delightful journey.

Detailed recipes

Recipe 1: Strawberry-Rhubarb Crumble

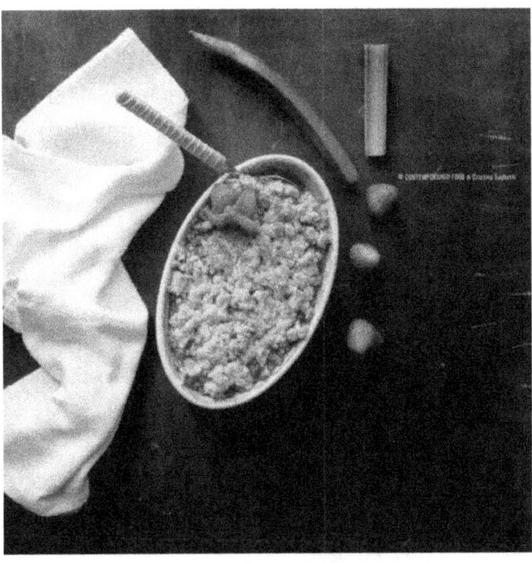

- **P. T. :** 20 minutes
- **Ingr. :** 3 cups diced strawberries, 1 cup diced rhubarb, 1/4 cup maple syrup, 1 cup oats, 1/2 cup almond flour, 1/4 cup melted coconut oil, 1/4 teaspoon cinnamon, pinch of salt.
- **Serv. :** Serves 6
- **M. of C. :** Baking
- **Process:**
    1. Preheat your oven to 375 degrees Fahrenheit.
    2. In a bowl, combine the strawberries, rhubarb, and maple syrup.
    3. Pour the fruit mixture into a baking dish.
    4. In a separate bowl, combine the oats, almond flour, coconut oil, cinnamon, and salt.
    5. Spread the crumble mixture over the fruit.

6. Bake for 25-30 minutes, or until the fruit is bubbling and the crumble is golden.

- **N. V. :**Per Serving: Calories: 252, Carbs: 32g, Protein: 5g, Fat: 12g, Fiber: 5g, Sugar: 15g

Recipe 2: Chocolate Avocado Mousse

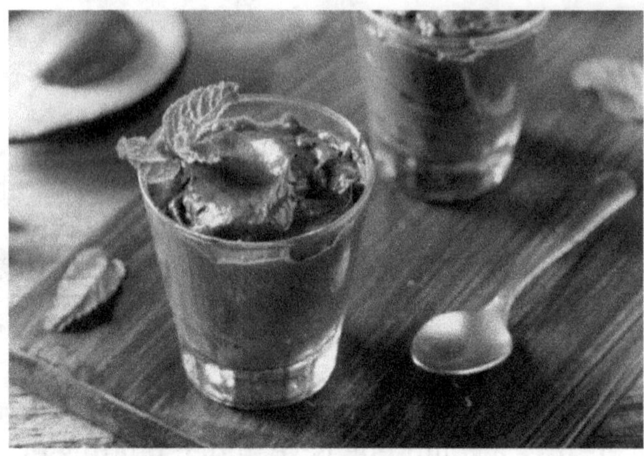

- **P. T. :** 10 minutes
- **Ingr. :**2 ripe avocados, 1/4 cup raw cacao powder, 1/4 cup maple syrup, 1 teaspoon vanilla extract, a pinch of salt.
- **Serv. :**Serves 4
- **M. of C. :**Blending
- **Process:**
    1. Scoop out the avocados and put them into a blender.
    2. Add the cacao powder, maple syrup, vanilla extract, and salt.
    3. Blend until smooth.
    4. Spoon the mousse into serving dishes and chill for at least an hour before serving.
- **N. V. :**Per Serving: Calories: 233, Carbs: 21g, Protein: 3g, Fat: 18g, Fiber: 7g, Sugar: 12g

Recipe 3: Blueberry Lemon Chia Pudding

- **P. T. :** 15 minutes
- **Ingr. :**1/4 cup chia seeds, 1 cup almond milk, 1 tablespoon lemon juice, 1 tablespoon maple syrup, 1/2 cup blueberries.
- **Serv. :**Serves 2
- **M. of C. :** No cook
- **Process:**
    1. Mix the chia seeds, almond milk, lemon juice, and maple syrup in a bowl.
    2. Let the mixture sit for about 10 minutes, until it thickens.
    3. Stir in the blueberries.
    4. Divide the pudding between two bowls and refrigerate for at least an hour before serving.
- **N. V. :**Per Serving: Calories: 185, Carbs: 26g, Protein: 5g, Fat: 8g, Fiber: 9g, Sugar: 11g

Recipe 4: Raspberry Coconut Bars

- **P. T. :** 25 minutes
- **Ingr. :**1 cup almond flour, 1/4 cup melted coconut oil, 1 tablespoon maple syrup, 1 cup raspberry jam, 1 cup shredded unsweetened coconut.
- **Serv. :**Makes 16 bars
- **M. of C. :**Baking
- **Process:**
    1. Preheat your oven to 350 degrees Fahrenheit.
    2. Mix the almond flour, coconut oil, and maple syrup to create a dough.
    3. Press the dough into the bottom of an 8x8 inch baking pan.

4. Spread the raspberry jam over the dough.
5. Sprinkle the shredded coconut on top.
6. Bake for 20-25 minutes, until the edges are golden.
7. Allow the bars to cool completely before cutting into squares.

- **N. V. :**Per Serving: Calories: 175, Carbs: 16g, Protein: 3g, Fat: 12g, Fiber: 3g, Sugar: 9g

Recipe 5: FODMAP Friendly Pavlova

- **P. T. :** 90 minutes
- **Ingr. :**4 egg whites, 1 cup sugar, 1 teaspoon white vinegar, 1/2 teaspoon cornstarch, 1/2 teaspoon vanilla extract, 1 cup lactose-free whipped cream, 2 cups strawberries.
- **Serv. :**Serves 6
- **M. of C. :**Baking
- **Process:**
    1. Preheat the oven to 250 degrees Fahrenheit and line a baking sheet with parchment paper.
    2. In a clean, dry bowl, beat egg whites until soft peaks form.
    3. Gradually add sugar, one tablespoon at a time, until the whites are stiff and shiny.
    4. Sprinkle vinegar, cornstarch, and vanilla extract over the egg whites and fold gently to combine.
    5. Spoon the mixture onto the prepared baking sheet and shape it into a circle.
    6. Bake for about 75 minutes or until the pavlova is dry to the touch.
    7. Turn off the oven and let the pavlova cool inside the oven.
    8. Once cooled, top with whipped cream and strawberries before serving.
- **N. V. :**Per Serving: Calories: 250, Carbs: 50g, Protein: 4g, Fat: 5g, Fiber: 1g, Sugar: 45g

Recipe 6: FODMAP Friendly Chocolate Chip Cookies

- **P. T. :** 30 minutes
- **Ingr. :**2 cups almond flour, 1/2 cup sugar, 1/2 cup dark chocolate chips, 1/2 cup melted coconut oil, 1/4 cup maple syrup, 1/2 teaspoon baking soda, 1/4 teaspoon salt.
- **Serv. :**Makes 12 cookies
- **M. of C. :**Baking
- **Process:**
    1. Preheat the oven to 350 degrees Fahrenheit and line a baking sheet with parchment paper.
    2. In a bowl, mix together the almond flour, sugar, chocolate chips, coconut oil, maple syrup, baking soda, and salt.
    3. Roll the dough into 12 balls and place them on the prepared baking sheet.
    4. Bake for about 10-12 minutes or until golden.
    5. Allow the cookies to cool on the baking sheet for 10 minutes before transferring to a wire rack to cool completely.
- **N. V. :**Per Serving: Calories: 265, Carbs: 23g, Protein: 5g, Fat: 18g, Fiber: 3g, Sugar: 17g

Recipe 7: FODMAP Friendly Rice Pudding

- **P. T. :** 60 minutes
- **Ingr. :**3/4 cup Arborio rice, 1/4 cup sugar, 4 cups lactose-free milk, 1/2 teaspoon vanilla extract, cinnamon to taste.
- **Serv. :**Serves 6
- **M. of C. :**Stovetop
- **Process:**
    1. In a large saucepan, combine rice, sugar, and milk.
    2. Bring to a boil, then reduce heat to low and simmer, stirring often, until rice is tender and creamy, about 45-50 minutes.
    3. Remove from heat and stir in vanilla extract.
    4. Let the pudding cool, then refrigerate until chilled. Sprinkle with cinnamon before serving.
- **N. V. :**Per Serving: Calories: 220, Carbs: 42g, Protein: 7g, Fat: 2.5g, Fiber: 1g, Sugar: 21g

Recipe 8: FODMAP Friendly Berry Sorbet

- **P. T. :** 10 minutes (plus freezing time)
- **Ingr. :**4 cups mixed berries (strawberries, blueberries, raspberries), 1/2 cup sugar, 1/4 cup water, 2 tablespoons lemon juice.
- **Serv. :**Serves 8
- **M. of C. :**Freezing
- **Process:**
    1. In a blender, puree the berries, sugar, water, and lemon juice until smooth.
    2. Strain the mixture through a fine-mesh sieve into a large bowl, discarding solids.
    3. Pour the mixture into a shallow dish and freeze for at least 4 hours or until firm.
    4. Before serving, let the sorbet soften at room temperature for 5-10 minutes.
- **N. V. :**Per Serving: Calories: 100, Carbs: 25g, Protein: 1g, Fat: 0g, Fiber: 3g, Sugar: 21g

Recipe 9: FODMAP Friendly Almond and Coconut Cookies

- **P. T. :** 30 minutes
- **Ingr. :**2 cups almond flour, 1/2 cup shredded unsweetened coconut, 1/2 cup maple syrup, 1/4 cup coconut oil, 1 tsp vanilla extract.
- **Serv. :**Makes 24 cookies
- **M. of C. :**Baking
- **Process:**
    1. Preheat the oven to 350°F (175°C). Line a baking sheet with parchment paper.
    2. Mix together the almond flour, shredded coconut, maple syrup, coconut oil, and vanilla extract in a large bowl.
    3. Roll the mixture into small balls, place on the baking sheet and flatten slightly.
    4. Bake for 15 minutes or until the edges are golden. Allow to cool completely before serving.
- **N. V. :**Per Serving: Calories: 106, Carbs: 8g, Protein: 2g, Fat: 8g, Fiber: 1g, Sugar: 6g

Recipe 10: FODMAP Friendly Vanilla Panna Cotta

- **P. T. :** 2 hours 20 minutes (including setting time)
- **Ingr. :**2 cups lactose-free cream, 1/4 cup sugar, 1 teaspoon gelatine, 1 teaspoon vanilla extract.

- **Serv. :**Serves 4
- **M. of C. :**Simmering
- **Process:**
    1. Sprinkle the gelatine over 1/4 cup of the cream and let it sit for 5 minutes.
    2. In a saucepan, heat the rest of the cream and sugar until the sugar dissolves.
    3. Remove from heat and stir in the gelatine and vanilla.
    4. Pour the mixture into four individual serving dishes and refrigerate for at least 2 hours or until set.
- **N. V. :**Per Serving: Calories: 314, Carbs: 15g, Protein: 3g, Fat: 27g, Fiber: 0g, Sugar: 15g

Recipe 11: FODMAP Friendly Pineapple and Mint Granita

- **P. T. :** 10 minutes (plus freezing time)
- **Ingr. :**1 ripe pineapple, peeled and cored, 1/4 cup sugar, 1/4 cup fresh mint leaves.
- **Serv. :**Serves 4
- **M. of C. :**Freezing
- **Process:**
    1. Puree the pineapple, sugar, and mint in a blender until smooth.
    2. Pour the mixture into a shallow dish and freeze until solid.
    3. Using a fork, scrape the frozen mixture to create flaky crystals. Serve immediately.
- **N. V. :**Per Serving: Calories: 110, Carbs: 29g, Protein: 1g, Fat: 0g, Fiber: 2g, Sugar: 25g

Recipe 12: FODMAP Friendly Lemon and Poppy Seed Loaf

- **P. T. :** 1 hour 15 minutes
- **Ingr. :**2 cups gluten-free flour blend, 1 cup sugar, 1/2 cup lactose-free milk, 1/2 cup vegetable oil, 2 large eggs, 2 tablespoons lemon zest, 2 tablespoons poppy seeds, 1 teaspoon baking powder, 1/2 teaspoon baking soda, 1/4 teaspoon salt.
- **Serv. :**Serves 10
- **M. of C. :**Baking
- **Process:**
    1. Preheat the oven to 350°F (175°C) and grease a loaf pan.
    2. In a large bowl, combine the flour, sugar, poppy seeds, baking powder, baking soda, and salt.
    3. In another bowl, whisk together the milk, oil, eggs, and lemon zest.
    4. Add the wet ingredients to the dry ingredients and mix until combined.
    5. Pour the batter into the prepared loaf pan and bake for 50-60 minutes or until a toothpick inserted into the center comes out clean.
    6. Allow to cool completely before slicing and serving.
- **N. V. :**Per Serving: Calories: 274, Carbs: 42g, Protein: 4g, Fat: 11g, Fiber: 3g, Sugar: 23g

Recipe 13: FODMAP Friendly Strawberry Sorbet

- **P. T. :** 4 hours 20 minutes (including freezing time)
- **Ingr. :**4 cups fresh strawberries, 1/2 cup sugar, 2 tablespoons lemon juice.

- **Serv. :**Serves 6
- **M. of C. :**Freezing
- **Process:**
    1. Blend the strawberries, sugar, and lemon juice until smooth.
    2. Strain the mixture through a sieve to remove the seeds.
    3. Pour the mixture into a shallow dish and freeze for 4 hours or until firm.
    4. Break the frozen mixture into chunks and blend again until smooth.
    5. Refreeze for another hour before serving.
- **N. V. :**Per Serving: Calories: 105, Carbs: 27g, Protein: 1g, Fat: 0g, Fiber: 2g, Sugar: 24g

Recipe 14: FODMAP Friendly Raspberry and Chocolate Chip Muffins

- **P. T. :** 40 minutes
- **Ingr. :**2 cups gluten-free flour blend, 1 cup sugar, 1/2 cup lactose-free milk, 1/2 cup vegetable oil, 2 large eggs, 1 cup fresh raspberries, 1/2 cup dark chocolate chips, 1 teaspoon baking powder, 1/2 teaspoon baking soda, 1/4 teaspoon salt.
- **Serv. :**Makes 12 muffins
- **M. of C. :**Baking
- **Process:**
    1. Preheat the oven to 350°F (175°C) and line a muffin tin with paper liners.
    2. In a large bowl, combine the flour, sugar, baking powder, baking soda, and salt.
    3. In another bowl, whisk together the milk, oil, and eggs.
    4. Add the wet ingredients to the dry ingredients and mix until combined.
    5. Gently fold in the raspberries and chocolate chips.
    6. Divide the batter among the muffin cups and bake for 20-25 minutes or until a toothpick inserted into the center comes out clean.
    7. Allow to cool in the pan for 10 minutes, then transfer to a wire rack to cool completely.
- **N. V. :**Per Muffin: Calories: 240, Carbs: 38g, Protein: 4g, Fat: 10g, Fiber: 3g, Sugar: 19g

Recipe 15: FODMAP Friendly Almond and Apricot Tart

- **P. T. :** 1 hour 10 minutes
- **Ingr. :**1 cup almond flour, 1/2 cup gluten-free flour blend, 1/2 cup sugar, 1/2 cup lactose-free butter, 1/2 cup almond milk, 2 large eggs, 1 cup fresh apricots, halved, 1 teaspoon almond extract, 1/2 teaspoon baking powder, 1/4 teaspoon salt.
- **Serv. :**Serves 8
- **M. of C. :**Baking
- **Process:**
    1. Preheat the oven to 350°F (175°C) and grease a tart pan.
    2. In a large bowl, combine the almond flour, gluten-free flour, baking powder, and salt.
    3. In another bowl, cream together the butter and sugar until light and fluffy.
    4. Beat in the eggs one at a time, followed by the almond extract.
    5. Gradually add the flour mixture, alternating with the almond milk, beginning and ending with the flour mixture.

6. Spread the batter in the prepared tart pan and arrange the apricot halves on top.
7. Bake for 40-45 minutes or until a toothpick inserted into the center comes out clean.
8. Allow to cool completely before slicing and serving.

- **N. V. :**Per Serving: Calories: 299, Carbs: 31g, Protein: 6g, Fat: 18g, Fiber: 3g, Sugar: 17g

Recipe 16: Low FODMAP Lemon Poppy Seed Cookies

- **P. T. :** 30 minutes
- **Ingr. :**2 cups gluten-free flour blend, 1 cup sugar, 1/2 cup lactose-free butter, 1 large egg, 2 tablespoons lemon juice, 2 teaspoons poppy seeds, 1 teaspoon baking powder, 1/2 teaspoon salt, Zest of 1 lemon.
- **Serv. :**Makes 24 cookies
- **M. of C. :**Baking
- **Process:**
    1. Preheat the oven to 350°F (175°C) and line two baking sheets with parchment paper.
    2. In a large bowl, combine the flour, sugar, baking powder, salt, and lemon zest.
    3. In another bowl, cream together the butter, egg, and lemon juice.
    4. Gradually add the dry ingredients to the wet ingredients, mixing until combined.
    5. Stir in the poppy seeds.
    6. Drop tablespoons of dough onto the prepared baking sheets and bake for 12-15 minutes or until lightly golden.
    7. Allow to cool on the baking sheets for 5 minutes, then transfer to a wire rack to cool completely.
- **N. V. :**Per Cookie: Calories: 110, Carbs: 18g, Protein: 1g, Fat: 4g, Fiber: 1g, Sugar: 9g

Recipe 17: FODMAP Friendly Banana Bread

- **P. T. :** 1 hour 15 minutes
- **Ingr. :**2 cups gluten-free flour blend, 1 cup sugar, 1/2 cup lactose-free butter, 2 large eggs, 4 ripe bananas, mashed, 1 teaspoon baking soda, 1/2 teaspoon salt.
- **Serv. :**Serves 10
- **M. of C. :**Baking
- **Process:**
    1. Preheat the oven to 350°F (175°C) and grease a loaf pan.
    2. In a large bowl, combine the flour, sugar, baking soda, and salt.
    3. In another bowl, cream together the butter and eggs.
    4. Add the mashed bananas to the wet ingredients and mix until combined.
    5. Gradually add the dry ingredients to the wet ingredients, mixing until combined.
    6. Pour the batter into the prepared loaf pan and bake for 60-65 minutes or until a toothpick inserted into the center comes out clean.
    7. Allow to cool in the pan for 10 minutes, then transfer to a wire rack to cool completely.

- **N. V. :**Per Serving: Calories: 271,
  Carbs: 46g, Protein: 4g, Fat: 9g,
  Fiber: 3g, Sugar: 23g

Recipe 18: Low FODMAP Vanilla Panna Cotta

- **P. T. :** 4 hours 10 minutes (including chilling time)
- **Ingr. :**2 cups lactose-free heavy cream, 1/2 cup sugar, 1 tablespoon gelatin, 2 teaspoons vanilla extract.
- **Serv. :**Serves 4
- **M. of C. :**Chilling
- **Process:**
  1. In a saucepan, combine the heavy cream and sugar and heat over medium heat until the sugar is dissolved.
  2. Sprinkle the gelatin over the cream mixture and stir until the gelatin is completely dissolved.
  3. Remove from the heat and stir in the vanilla extract.
  4. Divide the mixture among four ramekins and refrigerate for at least 4 hours or until set.
  5. Serve chilled.
- **N. V. :**Per Serving: Calories: 407, Carbs: 26g, Protein: 4g, Fat: 33g, Fiber: 0g, Sugar: 23g

Recipe 19: Low FODMAP Chocolate Fondant

- **P. T. :** 30 minutes
- **Ingr. :**1/2 cup lactose-free butter, 3/4 cup dark chocolate chips, 1/2 cup sugar, 2 large eggs, 1/4 cup cocoa powder, 1/4 cup gluten-free flour blend.
- **Serv. :**Serves 6
- **M. of C. :**Baking
- **Process:**
  1. Preheat the oven to 400°F (200°C) and grease six ramekins.
  2. Melt the butter and chocolate chips in a microwave or double boiler until smooth.
  3. In a separate bowl, beat together the sugar and eggs until pale and creamy.
  4. Fold the chocolate mixture, cocoa powder, and flour into the egg mixture until combined.
  5. Divide the mixture among the ramekins and bake for 12-15 minutes or until the edges are set but the center is still soft.
  6. Allow to cool for a few minutes, then serve warm.
- **N. V. :**Per Serving: Calories: 365, Carbs: 34g, Protein: 5g, Fat: 24g, Fiber: 3g, Sugar: 25g

Recipe 20: Low FODMAP Raspberry Almond Tart

- **P. T. :** 1 hour 30 minutes
- **Ingr. :**1 cup gluten-free flour blend, 1/2 cup ground almonds, 1/4 cup sugar, 1/2 cup lactose-free butter, 1/4 cup lactose-free milk, 1 cup fresh raspberries, 1/4 cup raspberry jam.
- **Serv. :**Serves 8
- **M. of C. :**Baking
- **Process:**
  1. Preheat the oven to 350°F (175°C) and grease a tart pan.
  2. In a large bowl, combine the flour, ground almonds, and sugar.

3. Cut in the butter until the mixture resembles coarse crumbs.
4. Gradually add the milk, stirring until a dough forms.
5. Press the dough into the bottom and up the sides of the prepared tart pan.
6. Bake for 15-20 minutes or until lightly golden.
7. Allow to cool, then spread the raspberry jam over the tart shell.
8. Arrange the raspberries on top of the jam.
9. Serve at room temperature.

- **N. V. :**Per Serving: Calories: 254, Carbs: 28g, Protein: 4g, Fat: 15g, Fiber: 3g, Sugar: 11g

Chapter 8: Beverages

Introduction

Welcome to the vibrant world of low FODMAP beverages! The variety of our carefully crafted drinks will not only hydrate but also rejuvenate your senses. Be it a comforting warm drink on a chilly day or a chilled refresher under the summer sun, these beverages are more than thirst-quenchers; they're health choices and lifestyle selections.

So, let's embark on this flavorful journey through a range of low FODMAP beverages. Manage your health and enjoy the taste of these delicious drinks. Welcome to the world of low FODMAP beverages!

Detailed recipes

Recipe 1: Ginger Infused Lemonade

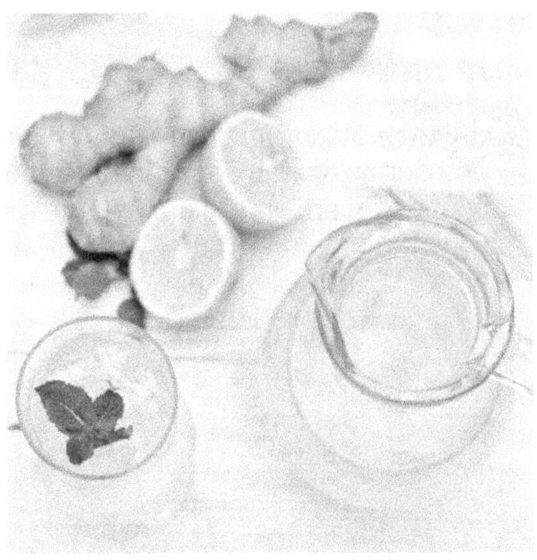

- **P. T. :** 15 min

- **Ingr. :**1 cup freshly squeezed lemon juice, 4 cups water, 1/2 cup sugar, 1 tablespoon freshly grated ginger, lemon slices, and ice cubes.
- **Serv. :**Serves 6
- **M. of C. :** Stovetop
- **Process:**Combine the sugar and 1 cup water in a saucepan over medium heat. Stir until the sugar dissolves, then add the ginger and simmer for 5 minutes. Allow it to cool and strain out the ginger. Mix this syrup with the lemon juice and remaining water. Serve over ice with lemon slices.
- **N. V. :**Each serving has 80 calories, 0.2g fat, 20.8g carbohydrates, 0.2g protein.

Recipe 2: Almond Milk Chai Latte

- **P. T. :** 10 min
- **Ingr. :**2 cups almond milk, 2 chai tea bags, 1 tablespoon honey, and a sprinkle of cinnamon.
- **Serv. :**Serves 2
- **M. of C. :** Stovetop
- **Process:**Heat the almond milk in a pot until hot but not boiling. Add the

chai tea bags and let them steep for 5 minutes. Remove the tea bags, stir in the honey, and serve with a sprinkle of cinnamon on top.

- **N. V. :**Each serving has 80 calories, 2.5g fat, 13g carbohydrates, 1g protein.

Recipe 3: Strawberry Kiwi Smoothie

- **P. T. :** 5 min
- **Ingr. :**2 cups fresh strawberries, 2 peeled kiwis, 1 cup non-fat Greek yogurt, and 1 cup ice.
- **Serv. :**Serves 2
- **M. of C. :** Blending
- **Process:**Blend all ingredients until smooth. Pour into glasses and serve immediately.
- **N. V. :**Each serving has 150 calories, 0.5g fat, 31g carbohydrates, 9g protein.

Recipe 4: Tropical Pineapple and Mango Juice

- **P. T. :** 10 min
- **Ingr. :**2 cups pineapple chunks, 1 cup peeled and chopped mango, and 1 cup ice.
- **Serv. :**Serves 2
- **M. of C. :** Juicing
- **Process:**Juice the pineapple and mango. Pour over ice and serve immediately.
- **N. V. :**Each serving has 120 calories, 0.3g fat, 30g carbohydrates, 1.2g protein.

Recipe 5: Golden Turmeric Latte

- **P. T. :** 10 min
- **Ingr. :**2 cups almond milk, 1 teaspoon turmeric, 1/2 teaspoon cinnamon, 1/4 teaspoon ginger powder, and 1 teaspoon honey.
- **Serv. :**Serves 2
- **M. of C. :** Stovetop
- **Process:**Heat the almond milk in a pot until hot but not boiling. Stir in the turmeric, cinnamon, and ginger powder until well combined. Remove from heat, stir in the honey, and serve warm.
- **N. V. :**Each serving has 70 calories, 2.5g fat, 10g carbohydrates, 1g protein.

Recipe 6: Green Goddess Smoothie

- **P. T. :** 5 min
- **Ingr. :**1 banana, 1 cup spinach, 1/2 avocado, 1 cup almond milk, and 1 tablespoon chia seeds.
- **Serv. :**Serves 1
- **M. of C. :** Blending
- **Process:**Blend all ingredients until smooth. Pour into a glass and serve immediately.
- **N. V. :**The serving has 350 calories, 19g fat, 40g carbohydrates, 10g protein.

Recipe 7: Fruity Iced Tea

- **P. T. :** 10 min
- **Ingr. :** 4 black tea bags, 4 cups boiling water, 1 cup apple juice, 1 orange (sliced), and ice.
- **Serv. :** Serves 4
- **M. of C. :** Steeping and chilling
- **Process:** Steep the tea bags in the boiling water for 5 minutes. Remove the tea bags and stir in the apple juice. Chill in the refrigerator. Serve over ice with a slice of orange.
- **N. V. :** Each serving has 30 calories, 0g fat, 8g carbohydrates, 0g protein.

Recipe 8: Spicy Tomato Juice

- **P. T. :** 10 min
- **Ingr. :** 4 cups tomato juice, 1/4 teaspoon salt, 1/4 teaspoon black pepper, 1/4 teaspoon cayenne pepper, juice of 1 lemon.
- **Serv. :** Serves 4
- **M. of C. :** Mixing
- **Process:** Combine all ingredients in a pitcher and stir well to combine. Chill in the refrigerator for at least an hour before serving.
- **N. V. :** Each serving has 50 calories, 0g fat, 12g carbohydrates, 2g protein.

Recipe 9: Berry Bliss Smoothie

- **P. T. :** 5 min
- **Ingr. :** 1 cup frozen mixed berries, 1 banana, 1 cup almond milk, 1 tablespoon chia seeds.
- **Serv. :** Serves 1
- **M. of C. :** Blending
- **Process:** Blend all ingredients until smooth. Pour into a glass and serve immediately.
- **N. V. :** The serving has 300 calories, 8g fat, 50g carbohydrates, 8g protein.

Recipe 10: Minty Iced Green Tea

- **P. T. :** 15 min
- **Ingr. :** 4 green tea bags, 4 cups boiling water, 1/4 cup fresh mint leaves, 1 tablespoon honey, ice.
- **Serv. :** Serves 4
- **M. of C. :** Steeping and chilling
- **Process:** Steep the tea bags and mint leaves in the boiling water for 5 minutes. Remove the tea bags and mint leaves and stir in the honey. Chill in the refrigerator. Serve over ice.
- **N. V. :** Each serving has 25 calories, 0g fat, 7g carbohydrates, 0g protein.

Recipe 11: Soothing Chamomile Honey Tea

- **P. T. :** 10 min
- **Ingr. :** 2 chamomile tea bags, 2 cups boiling water, 2 teaspoons honey.
- **Serv. :** Serves 2
- **M. of C. :** Steeping
- **Process:** Steep the chamomile tea bags in the boiling water for 5 minutes. Remove the tea bags and stir in the honey until dissolved. Serve warm.
- **N. V. :** Each serving has 30 calories, 0g fat, 8g carbohydrates, 0g protein.

Recipe 12: Cool Cucumber Water

- **P. T. :** 5 min
- **Ingr. :**1 cucumber, 8 cups cold water.
- **Serv. :**Serves 8
- **M. of C. :** Infusing
- **Process:**Slice the cucumber thinly. Add cucumber slices to the water and refrigerate for at least 1 hour before serving.
- **N. V. :**Each serving has 5 calories, 0g fat, 1g carbohydrates, 0g protein.

Recipe 13: Citrus Ginger Fizz

- **P. T. :** 5 min
- **Ingr. :**1 cup freshly squeezed orange juice, 1 teaspoon grated ginger, 1 cup sparkling water.
- **Serv. :**Serves 1
- **M. of C. :** Mixing
- **Process:**Combine orange juice and grated ginger in a glass. Top with sparkling water and stir gently. Serve chilled.
- **N. V. :**The serving has 110 calories, 0g fat, 26g carbohydrates, 2g protein.

Recipe 14: Fresh Mint Iced Tea

- **P. T. :** 15 min
- **Ingr. :**4 green tea bags, 4 cups boiling water, 1 cup fresh mint leaves, ice cubes.
- **Serv. :**Serves 4
- **M. of C. :** Steeping
- **Process:**Steep the tea bags and mint leaves in the boiling water for 10 minutes. Remove the tea bags and mint, then chill in the refrigerator. Serve over ice.
- **N. V. :**Each serving has 2 calories, 0g fat, 0.5g carbohydrates, 0g protein.

Recipe 15: Blueberry Smoothie

- **P. T. :** 5 min
- **Ingr. :**1 cup fresh blueberries, 1 banana, 1/2 cup Greek yogurt, 1 cup almond milk.
- **Serv. :**Serves 2
- **M. of C. :** Blending
- **Process:**Combine all ingredients in a blender and blend until smooth. Serve immediately.
- **N. V. :**Each serving has 150 calories, 2g fat, 30g carbohydrates, 6g protein.

Recipe 16: Warm Apple Cider

- **P. T. :** 15 min
- **Ingr. :**4 cups apple cider, 2 cinnamon sticks, 4 cloves.
- **Serv. :**Serves 4
- **M. of C. :** Heating
- **Process:**Combine all ingredients in a pot and simmer for 10 minutes. Strain and serve hot.
- **N. V. :**Each serving has 120 calories, 0g fat, 30g carbohydrates, 0g protein.

Recipe 17: Coconut Water Smoothie

- **P. T. :** 10 min
- **Ingr. :** 2 cups fresh pineapple, 1 cup coconut water, 1 cup ice, 1 tbsp honey.
- **Serv. :** Serves 2
- **M. of C. :** Blending
- **Process:** Combine all ingredients in a blender and blend until smooth. Serve immediately.
- **N. V. :** Each serving has 100 calories, 0g fat, 26g carbohydrates, 1g protein.

Recipe 18: Raspberry Lemonade

- **P. T. :** 20 min
- **Ingr. :** 1 cup fresh raspberries, 1 cup fresh lemon juice, 1/2 cup sugar, 4 cups water.
- **Serv. :** Serves 4
- **M. of C. :** Blending and Mixing
- **Process:** Blend the raspberries until smooth, then strain to remove seeds. Mix the raspberry juice, lemon juice, sugar, and water in a pitcher until sugar is dissolved. Chill and serve over ice.
- **N. V. :** Each serving has 80 calories, 0g fat, 21g carbohydrates, 0g protein.

Recipe 19: Iced Latte

- **P. T. :** 10 min
- **Ingr. :** 2 shots of espresso, 1 cup cold milk, 1 tsp sugar, ice cubes.
- **Serv. :** Serves 1
- **M. of C. :** Mixing
- **Process:** Mix the espresso shots with sugar until dissolved. Fill a glass with ice, pour the sweetened espresso over it, and top with milk. Serve immediately.
- **N. V. :** The serving has 100 calories, 2g fat, 13g carbohydrates, 6g protein.

Recipe 20: Cucumber Lime Water

- **P. T. :** 10 min
- **Ingr. :** 1 cucumber, sliced, 2 limes, sliced, 4 cups water.
- **Serv. :** Serves 4
- **M. of C. :** Infusing
- **Process:** Combine all ingredients in a pitcher and refrigerate for at least an hour before serving to allow flavors to infuse.
- **N. V. :** Each serving has 15 calories, 0g fat, 4g carbohydrates, 1g protein.

Chapter 9: Sauces, Dressings, and Condiments

Introduction to Sauces, Dressings, and Condiments

Chapter 9 dives into the rich, tantalizing world of sauces, dressings, and condiments. These elements, often overlooked, are the hidden champions that can transform a simple dish into a gastronomic delight. This section aims to inspire the urban dweller, whether you're a fitness-conscious male in his thirties or a career-oriented woman looking to enhance her family's diet. The exploration of these recipes isn't just about satiating taste buds, but about embracing a dietary approach that caters to specific health needs, including managing IBS symptoms or enriching nutritional knowledge for personal or professional growth. It's about crafting homemade culinary gems that pack a flavorful punch, and simultaneously, adhere to the Low-FODMAP guidelines. Let's embark on this flavorful journey together, adding a little extra zest to our meals, and a lot more health to our lives.

Detailed recipes

Recipe 1: Tangy FODMAP-friendly Tomato Sauce

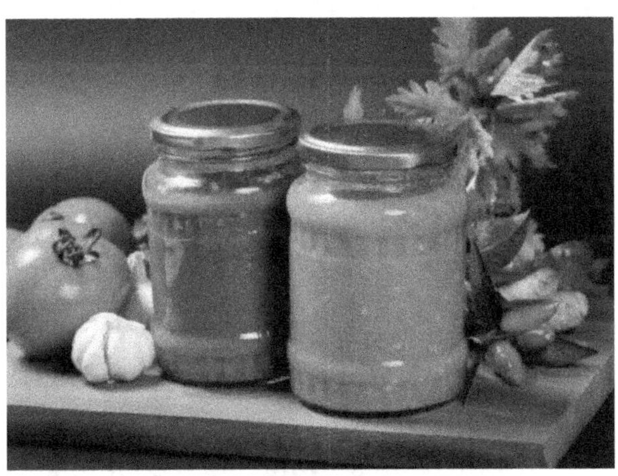

- **P. T. :**15 mins
- **Ingr. :**1 cup canned tomatoes (low FODMAP certified), 1 tablespoon garlic-infused oil, 1/2 teaspoon dried basil, 1/2 teaspoon dried oregano, salt and pepper to taste.
- **Serv. :** 4
- M. of Prep. : Stovetop
- **Process:**Heat the garlic-infused oil in a pan over medium heat. Add canned tomatoes, dried basil, dried oregano, salt, and pepper. Let it simmer for 10 minutes, stirring occasionally.
- **N. V. :**Kcal42, Total Fat 3.5g, Sodium 283mg, Total Carbohydrate 3g, Dietary Fiber 1g, Sugars 2g, Protein 1g.

Recipe 2: Zesty Lemon Vinaigrette

- P. T. :5 mins

- **Ingr. :**1/4 cup lemon juice, 1/2 cup olive oil, 2 tablespoons maple syrup, salt, and pepper to taste.
- **Serv. :** 8
- M. of Prep. : Whisking
- **Process:**In a bowl, whisk together all the ingredients until well combined.
- **N. V. :**Kcal123, Total Fat 13.5g, Sodium 1mg, Total Carbohydrate 3g, Sugars 3g.

Recipe 3: Spicy Salsa Verde

- **P. T. :**15 mins
- **Ingr. :**2 cups chopped green tomatoes, 1/2 cup chopped scallions (green part only), 1 jalapeno, 2 tablespoons lime juice, salt to taste.
- **Serv. :** 4
- M. of Prep. : Blending
- **Process:**Add all ingredients to a blender and blend until smooth.
- **N. V. :**Kcal30, Total Fat 0.3g, Sodium 9mg, Total Carbohydrate 7g, Dietary Fiber 2g, Sugars 4g, Protein 1g.

Recipe 4: Creamy Garlic-Infused Aioli

- **P. T. :**10 mins
- **Ingr. :**1 cup mayonnaise, 2 tablespoons garlic-infused oil, 1 tablespoon lemon juice, salt to taste.
- **Serv. :** 16
- M. of Prep. : Whisking
- **Process:**In a bowl, whisk together all the ingredients until smooth.
- **N. V. :**Kcal94, Total Fat 10.3g, Sodium 75mg, Total Carbohydrate 0.1g.

Recipe 5: Low-FODMAP BBQ Sauce

- **P. T. :**20 mins
- **Ingr. :**1 cup canned tomatoes, 1/4 cup brown sugar, 2 tablespoons Worcestershire sauce (gluten-free), 1 tablespoon garlic-infused oil, 1 tablespoon apple cider vinegar, salt and pepper to taste.
- **Serv. :** 8
- M. of Prep. : Simmering
- **Process:**In a saucepan, combine all ingredients and simmer for 15 minutes until thickened.
- **N. V. :**Kcal58, Total Fat 1.7g, Sodium 73mg, Total Carbohydrate 10.8g, Sugars 9.5g.

Recipe 6: Asian-style Low-FODMAP Soy Sauce

- **P. T. :**5 mins
- **Ingr. :**1 cup of water, 2 tablespoons beef bouillon, 1 tablespoon balsamic vinegar, 1 tablespoon molasses, 1 teaspoon ginger-infused oil.
- **Serv. :** 16
- M. of Prep. : Mixing
- **Process:**Combine all ingredients in a bowl and stir until well combined.
- **N. V. :**Kcal10, Total Fat 0.6g, Sodium 70mg, Total Carbohydrate 1.2g, Sugars 1g.

Recipe 7: Classic Low-FODMAP Marinara Sauce

- **P. T. :**30 mins
- **Ingr. :**1 can (28 oz) of crushed tomatoes, 1 tablespoon garlic-infused

oil, 1 tablespoon sugar, 1 tablespoon basil, salt and pepper to taste.
- **Serv. :** 8
- M. of Prep. : Simmering
- **Process:**In a saucepan, heat the garlic-infused oil, add the crushed

tomatoes, sugar, basil, and season with salt and pepper. Simmer for 25-30 minutes.
- **N. V. :**Kcal46, Total Fat 1.4g, Sodium 13mg, Total Carbohydrate 8.3g, Sugars 5.3g.

Recipe 8: Tangy Raspberry Vinaigrette

- **P. T. :**10 mins
- **Ingr. :**1 cup fresh raspberries, 1/4 cup raspberry vinegar, 1/4 cup olive oil, 2 tablespoons maple syrup, salt and pepper to taste.
- **Serv. :** 8
- M. of Prep. : Blending
- **Process:**Combine all ingredients in a blender and blend until smooth. Strain to remove raspberry seeds if desired.
- **N. V. :**Kcal99, Total Fat 7g, Sodium 1mg, Total Carbohydrate 8.8g, Sugars 7.6g.

Recipe 9: Creamy Avocado Dressing

- **P. T. :**10 mins
- **Ingr. :**1 ripe avocado, 1/4 cup lime juice, 1/4 cup olive oil, salt and pepper to taste.
- **Serv. :** 8
- M. of Prep. : Blending
- **Process:**Combine all ingredients in a blender and blend until smooth.
- **N. V. :**Kcal106, Total Fat 10.6g, Sodium 2mg, Total Carbohydrate 3.8g, Dietary Fiber 2g, Sugars 0.6g.

Recipe 10: FODMAP-friendly Peanut Sauce

- **P. T. :**10 mins
- **Ingr. :**1/2 cup peanut butter, 2 tablespoons lime juice, 2 tablespoons soy sauce (gluten-free), 1 tablespoon brown sugar, 1 tablespoon ginger-infused oil.
- **Serv. :** 8
- M. of Prep. : Whisking
- **Process:**Whisk all ingredients in a bowl until smooth.
- **N. V. :**Kcal129, Total Fat 10.2g, Sodium 123mg, Total Carbohydrate 6.2g, Sugars 3.4g.

Recipe 11: Low-FODMAP Blue Cheese Dressing

- **P. T. :**10 mins
- **Ingr. :**1 cup lactose-free sour cream, 1/2 cup blue cheese crumbles, 2 tablespoons chives, 1 tablespoon lemon juice, salt and pepper to taste.
- **Serv. :** 10
- M. of Prep. : Mixing
- **Process:**Combine all ingredients in a bowl and stir until well combined. Chill before serving.
- **N. V. :**Kcal94, Total Fat 7.6g, Sodium 146mg, Total Carbohydrate 2.2g, Sugars 1.8g.

Recipe 12: Low-FODMAP Pesto Sauce

- **P. T. :**10 mins
- **Ingr. :**2 cups fresh basil leaves, 1/2 cup garlic-infused olive oil, 1/2 cup grated parmesan, 1/4 cup pine nuts, salt and pepper to taste.
- **Serv. :** 8
- M. of Prep. : Blending
- **Process:**Combine all ingredients in a blender or food processor and blend until smooth.
- **N. V. :**Kcal207, Total Fat 20.3g, Sodium 108mg, Total Carbohydrate 2.2g, Dietary Fiber 0.6g, Sugars 0.4g.

Recipe 13: Low-FODMAP Tartar Sauce

- **P. T. :**10 mins
- **Ingr. :**1 cup mayonnaise, 3 tablespoons dill pickles, 1 tablespoon fresh dill, 1 tablespoon capers, 1 teaspoon mustard.
- **Serv. :** 10
- M. of Prep. : Mixing
- **Process:**Combine all ingredients in a bowl and stir until well combined.
- **N. V. :**Kcal197, Total Fat 21.2g, Sodium 238mg, Total Carbohydrate 0.7g, Sugars 0.6g.

Recipe 14: Low-FODMAP Chimichurri Sauce

- **P. T. :**10 mins
- **Ingr. :**1 cup fresh parsley, 1/2 cup garlic-infused olive oil, 1/4 cup red wine vinegar, 1/4 teaspoon chili flakes, salt to taste.
- **Serv. :** 8
- M. of Prep. : Blending
- **Process:**Combine all ingredients in a blender or food processor and blend until smooth.
- **N. V. :**Kcal132, Total Fat 14g, Sodium 5mg, Total Carbohydrate 0.7g, Sugars 0.1g.

Recipe 15: Low-FODMAP Tomato Salsa

- **P. T. :**10 mins
- **Ingr. :**2 ripe tomatoes, 1/4 cup green bell pepper, 1/4 cup red bell pepper, 2 tablespoons fresh cilantro, 1 tablespoon lime juice, salt and pepper to taste.
- **Serv. :** 8
- M. of Prep. : Mixing
- **Process:**Chop all vegetables finely and combine in a bowl. Add lime juice, salt and pepper and stir well.
- **N. V. :**Kcal13, Total Fat 0.1g, Sodium 3mg, Total Carbohydrate 3g, Dietary Fiber 0.8g, Sugars 2g.

Recipe 16: Low-FODMAP Greek Vinaigrette

- **P. T. :**10 mins
- **Ingr. :**1/2 cup garlic-infused olive oil, 1/4 cup red wine vinegar, 1 teaspoon dried oregano, salt and pepper to taste.
- **Serv. :** 8
- M. of Prep. : Mixing
- **Process:**Whisk together all ingredients until well combined.
- **N. V. :**Kcal125, Total Fat 14g, Sodium 1mg, Total Carbohydrate 0.2g.

Recipe 17: Low-FODMAP Honey Mustard Sauce

- **P. T. :**10 mins

- **Ingr. :**1/2 cup Dijon mustard, 1/4 cup honey, 1/4 cup apple cider vinegar, 1/4 cup mayonnaise.
- **Serv. :** 8
- M. of Prep. : Mixing

- **Process:**Whisk together all ingredients until smooth.
- **N. V. :**Kcal126, Total Fat 7.2g, Sodium 230mg, Total Carbohydrate 15.8g, Sugars 14.3g.

Recipe 18: Low-FODMAP Barbecue Sauce

- **P. T. :**30 mins
- **Ingr. :**1 cup tomato passata, 1/2 cup brown sugar, 1/4 cup apple cider vinegar, 1 tablespoon Worcestershire sauce, 1 teaspoon smoked paprika, salt to taste.
- **Serv. :** 8

- M. of Prep. : Simmering
- **Process:**Combine all ingredients in a saucepan over medium heat. Simmer for 20 minutes or until thickened.
- **N. V. :**Kcal77, Total Fat 0.1g, Sodium 44mg, Total Carbohydrate 19.2g, Sugars 17.6g.

Recipe 19: Low-FODMAP Caesar Dressing

- **P. T. :**10 mins
- **Ingr. :**1 cup mayonnaise, 1/2 cup grated parmesan, 2 tablespoons lemon juice, 1 tablespoon Worcestershire sauce, salt and pepper to taste.
- **Serv. :** 8

- M. of Prep. : Mixing
- **Process:**Whisk together all ingredients until smooth.
- **N. V. :**Kcal209, Total Fat 20.7g, Sodium 225mg, Total Carbohydrate 1.9g, Sugars 1.3g.

Recipe 20: Low-FODMAP Marinara Sauce

- P. T. :1 hour
- **Ingr. :**2 cups canned tomatoes, 1/4 cup garlic-infused olive oil, 1 teaspoon dried basil, 1 teaspoon dried oregano, salt to taste.
- **Serv. :** 8
- M. of Prep. : Simmering

- **Process:**Combine all ingredients in a saucepan over medium heat. Simmer for 45 minutes or until sauce has thickened.
- **N. V. :** Kcal70, Total Fat 7g, Sodium 12mg, Total Carbohydrate 3.6g, Sugars 2.4g.

Chapter 10: 4-Week Meal Plan

Introduction to the Meal Plan

Charting your course towards better health starts with an effective, well-structured meal plan, especially if your goals include managing IBS symptoms, staying fit, enhancing your family's well-being, or learning about various diets.
We've chosen recipes that are quick, flavorful, and easy to prepare with readily available ingredients. They align with the low-FODMAP diet, making it easier for you to meet your goals without compromising on taste or variety.

Each week is further broken down into daily meal plans for better clarity and ease of use. Remember, a meal plan is a guide, not a rigid prescription. Feel free to swap out ingredients, experiment with flavors, and make each meal your own. Welcome to this 4-week journey of flavorful, healthful eating!

Week 1: Detailed daily meal plan

In this section, we dive into a detailed daily meal plan for Week 1.

Day	Breakfast	Lunch	Dinner	Snacks/Appetizers	Dessert	Beverage	Condiment
Day 1	Buckwheat Pancakes with Berries	Garden Vegetable Quinoa Salad	Lemon and Dill Salmon	Roasted Chickpeas	Mango Sorbet	Green Detox Juice	Garlic-infused Olive Oil
Day 2	Vegetable and Tofu Scramble	Chicken Caesar Wrap	Quinoa Stuffed Bell Peppers	Carrot and Cucumber Sticks with Hummus	Strawberry and Banana Smoothie Bowl	Pomegranate and Mint Infused Water	Low-FODMAP Marinara Sauce
Day 3	Spinach and Egg Muffins	Grilled Tuna with Olive Tapenade	Chicken and Eggplant Curry	Bell Pepper and Cucumber Crudité with Hummus	Dark Chocolate Dipped Strawberries	Blueberry and Basil Infused Water	Low-FODMAP BBQ Sauce
Day 4	Quinoa Breakfast Bowl with Berries	Asian Chicken Salad	Beef and Vegetable Stir-fry	Roasted Pumpkin Seeds	Gluten-free Apple Crumble	Pineapple and Mint Infused Water	Low-FODMAP Pesto
Day 5	Oatmeal with Blueberries and Chia Seeds	Roasted Vegetable Quinoa Salad	Baked Cod with Lemon and Dill	Baked Potato Chips	Berry and Banana Smoothie Bowl	Lemon and Ginger Infused Water	Maple Mustard Dressing
Day 6	Almond Flour Pancakes with Maple Syrup	Greek-style Chicken Wraps	Baked Risotto with Roasted Vegetables	Cherry Tomatoes with Mozzarella Balls	Raspberry Sorbet	Watermelon and Basil Infused Water	Low-FODMAP Salsa

Week 2: Detailed daily meal plan

In this section, we dive into a detailed daily meal plan for Week 2.

Day	Breakfast	Lunch	Dinner	Snacks/Appetizers	Dessert	Beverage	Condiment
Day 1	Smoothie Bowl with Mixed Berries	Tuna Salad with a Twist	Quinoa with Grilled Shrimp	Veggie Sticks with Avocado Hummus	Coconut Milk Ice Cream	Infused Water with Citrus Fruits	Low-FODMAP Guacamole
Day 2	Scrambled Tofu with Mixed Vegetables	Turkey Wrap with Gluten-Free Tortilla	Salmon with Sweet Potato Mash	Rice Cakes with Almond Butter	Berry Parfait with Coconut Yogurt	Green Detox Smoothie	Low-FODMAP Teriyaki Sauce
Day 3	Buckwheat Porridge with Apple	Grilled Chicken with Quinoa Salad	Eggplant Lasagna	Assorted Nuts and Seeds	Chocolate-dipped Strawberries	Lemon and Cucumber Infused Water	Low-FODMAP Tomato Sauce
Day 4	Rice Cakes with Avocado	Vegan Sushi Rolls	Beef Stir-fry with Bell Peppers	Carrot and Cucumber Sticks with Hummus	Banana and Strawberry Sorbet	Pineapple and Ginger Infused Water	Low-FODMAP Salsa
Day 5	Smoothie with Banana, Spinach and Chia Seeds	Tofu Stir-fry with Vegetables	Baked Chicken with Zucchini Noodles	Cherry Tomatoes with Mozzarella Balls	Lemon and Blueberry Frozen Yogurt	Infused Water with Berries	Low-FODMAP Pesto
Day 6	Almond Flour Waffles with Berries	Vegan Buddha Bowl	Spaghetti Squash with Marinara Sauce	Vegetable Crudités with Garlic-infused Olive Oil	Dark Chocolate Almond Butter Cups	Green Juice with Spinach and Apple	Low-FODMAP BBQ Sauce

Week 3: Detailed daily meal plan

In this section, we dive into a detailed daily meal plan for Week 3.

Day	Breakfast	Lunch	Dinner	Snacks/Appetizers	Dessert	Beverage	Condiment
Day 1	Chia Pudding with Mixed Berries	Gluten-Free Chicken Quesadilla	Zoodles with Pesto and Shrimp	Greek Salad Bites	Dark Chocolate Covered Bananas	Infused Water with Lemon and Mint	Low-FODMAP Marinara Sauce
Day 2	Quinoa Porridge with Cinnamon and Apple	Vegetable Stir-fry with Tofu	Grilled Salmon with Dill Sauce	Mini Rice Cake Sandwiches	Lemon Sorbet with Berries	Herbal Tea	Low-FODMAP Caesar Dressing
Day 3	Gluten-Free Toast with Avocado and Tomatoes	Sushi Bowl with Salmon	Veggie-loaded Pizza on Gluten-free Crust	Veggie Sticks with Hummus	Raspberry Coconut Milk Ice Cream	Green Smoothie	Low-FODMAP Sweet and Sour Sauce
Day 4	Veggie Omelette with Chives	Shrimp Salad with Lemon Vinaigrette	Baked Chicken with Steamed Vegetables	Fruit Salad with a drizzle of Honey	Chocolate Avocado Mousse	Infused Water with Berries	Low-FODMAP Vinaigrette
Day 5	Buckwheat Pancakes with Maple Syrup	Quinoa Salad with Grilled Veggies	Beef Tacos with Gluten-Free Tortillas	Assorted Olives and Pickles	Baked Apples with Cinnamon	Fresh Orange Juice	Low-FODMAP Garlic Infused Oil

Week 4: Detailed daily meal plan

In this section, we dive into a detailed daily meal plan for Week 4.

Day	Breakfast	Lunch	Dinner	Snacks/Appetizers	Dessert	Beverage	Condiment
Day 1	Blueberry Oatmeal with Chia Seeds	Quinoa Salad with Grilled Chicken	Grilled Tofu with Stir-fried Veggies	Spicy Roasted Chickpeas	Avocado Chocolate Pudding	Infused Water with Cucumber and Mint	Low-FODMAP BBQ Sauce
Day 2	Avocado Smoothie with Spinach and Pineapple	Shrimp Stir-fry with Bell Peppers	Beef and Vegetable Curry	Rice Cakes with Almond Butter	Gluten-free Chocolate Chip Cookies	Green Tea	Low-FODMAP Teriyaki Sauce
Day 3	Gluten-free Waffles with Berries	Zucchini Noodles with Lemon-Garlic Shrimp	Baked Chicken with Steamed Broccoli	Fresh Vegetable Sticks with Guacamole	Strawberry Banana Sorbet	Herbal Tea	Low-FODMAP Pesto Sauce
Day 4	Smoothie Bowl with Berries and Seeds	Gluten-free Chicken Wrap	Baked Salmon with Dill and Lemon	Assorted Nuts and Seeds	Dark Chocolate Dipped Strawberries	Freshly Squeezed Orange Juice	Low-FODMAP Salsa
Day 5	Scrambled Eggs with Spinach	Tofu Salad with Ginger-Soy Dressing	Quinoa Stuffed Bell Peppers	Greek Salad Skewers	Baked Pears with Honey and Cinnamon	Infused Water with Berries	Low-FODMAP Ranch Dressing
Day 6	Quinoa Porridge with Apples and Cinnamon	Vegetable Soup with Quinoa	Grilled Steak with Sweet Potato Fries	Fruit Salad with a Drizzle of Honey	Blueberry Almond Crumble	Iced Green Tea	Low-FODMAP Garlic Infused Oil

Chapter 11: Eating Out and Traveling on a Low-FODMAP Diet

Tips for Dining Out

Navigating the dining scene while adhering to a Low-FODMAP diet can feel like charting unexplored territory. However, equipped with the right tools and mindset, you'll soon become a maestro of managing your menu choices, turning dining out from a challenge into an enjoyable experience.

Choosing a Restaurant

Finding a restaurant that caters to a Low-FODMAP diet does not have to feel like searching for a needle in a haystack. In this digital era, a quick online search or glance at an app can provide insights into a restaurant's offerings. Reading through the menu beforehand allows you to determine whether a restaurant has Low-FODMAP friendly options. Opt for places that highlight fresh, unprocessed foods and offer flexibility in their menu.

However, it's not just about the food. Consider the ambience too. An environment that allows you to relax and enjoy your meal can alleviate stress, which may help minimize IBS symptoms.

What to Order

Choosing what to order from the menu is akin to directing your food symphony. Start with a simple base; foods you know are safe for you. Plain meats, seafood, poultry, or tofu are good starting points. The same applies to the choice of vegetables and grains, provided they are cooked in a Low-FODMAP manner.

Substitution is your secret weapon. Swap high-FODMAP ingredients with those friendly to your diet. This simple maneuver can make most dishes Low-FODMAP appropriate.

Equally important is the way food is prepared. Grilled, steamed, or roasted foods are generally safer choices than fried or creamy dishes. If you are unsure about an item, do not hesitate to ask. Communication with the restaurant staff about your dietary restrictions will help them assist you better.

Remember, dining out is as much about the experience as it is about the food. Don't let your diet stop you from enjoying the ambiance, the company, and the joy that comes with trying new foods. After all, every culinary adventure is an opportunity for discovery and growth on your Low-FODMAP journey.

Packing Low-FODMAP Snacks for Travel

Travel and exploration are integral aspects of the human spirit, invigorating and enriching our lives in countless ways. However, for those following a Low-FODMAP diet, the uncertainty of what's available on the road can be daunting. But fear not, for packing Low-FODMAP snacks for travel can turn these uncertainties into opportunities for delicious culinary self-sufficiency.

Travel-Friendly Snack Ideas

Armed with an assortment of Low-FODMAP snacks, you can travel confidently, knowing that you have dependable options to keep your tummy content while you feed your wanderlust. Consider taking along hard cheese or lactose-free yoghurt for a protein kick, or rice cakes and gluten-free pretzels for a satisfying crunch. Fresh bananas, oranges, grapes, and strawberries can satisfy your sweet tooth, while homemade low-FODMAP granola bars or trail mix make for handy and nourishing nibbles during your journey.

But why limit ourselves to only the familiar? As adventurous travelers, let's push our culinary boundaries. Consider packing a jar of low-FODMAP salsa with corn chips, or even a small container of olives or pickles for a savory twist. With a little imagination, your travel snack pack can be as diverse and exciting as the destination you're heading to.

Packing Tips

The art of packing food for travel lies in maximizing freshness while minimizing bulk. Utilize resealable bags or containers to keep your snacks fresh and avoid unwanted spillages. Sturdy fruits like oranges and bananas can travel well without special packaging, while more delicate items like berries or cheese might require a bit more protection.

Insulated travel bags can help keep snacks cool and fresh, especially in warmer climates or long journeys. And remember, even non-perishable items like rice cakes or granola bars are best kept in air-tight containers to maintain their texture and taste.

In essence, travel does not have to disrupt your Low-FODMAP lifestyle. With a bit of planning and creative thinking, you can maintain your diet while experiencing the joy and discovery that comes with exploring new horizons. Remember, travel is a journey, and every journey is an opportunity to learn, grow, and enjoy the delicious diversity life has to offer.

Navigating International Cuisine

Embracing the flavors of different cultures is an inherent part of traveling. It's an opportunity to expand our culinary horizons and enjoy the taste tapestry of our global community. However, navigating international cuisine on a low-FODMAP diet can sometimes feel like deciphering a complex culinary cipher. Fear not, this guide will help demystify that process.

Common High-FODMAP Foods in Different Cuisines

Each cuisine is distinct, having evolved with its region's history, culture, and agricultural resources. This unique blend makes international dishes both exciting and sometimes challenging for those following a low-FODMAP diet. For instance, traditional Italian cuisine often features garlic and onions, both high in FODMAPs. Asian cuisines frequently use soy sauce and mushrooms, while many Mexican dishes are centered around beans and wheat tortillas.

Navigating these high-FODMAP ingredients doesn't mean you should shy away from international cuisines. Instead, think of it as an invitation to delve deeper into the culinary practices of the world, learning and appreciating the breadth and depth of ingredients and methods that each culture has to offer.

Tips for Eating Abroad

Eating abroad on a low-FODMAP diet is about finding balance. It's important to savor the unique flavors and traditions of the country you are in while also maintaining your health. Begin by learning a few phrases in the local language to communicate your dietary needs, or consider carrying a card that outlines them.

Asking about the ingredients and preparation methods is key. Opt for dishes that prioritize fresh, local produce, and lean meats. These often have fewer high-FODMAP ingredients. For instance, a Greek salad without onions or a simple grilled fish dish in Spain could work beautifully within your dietary needs.

Moreover, don't hesitate to explain your dietary restrictions at the restaurant. Many places are more than willing to adjust their dishes to accommodate their guests.

Navigating international cuisine while adhering to a low-FODMAP diet is more than feasible—it's a culinary adventure. It invites mindfulness and engagement with our food and its cultural context, enhancing the overall travel experience. So here's to a journey filled with culinary discoveries and gastronomic joy, all within the parameters of a diet that's kind to your body.

Chapter 12: Additional Resources

Websites, Blogs, and Apps for Low-FODMAP Living

Embracing a low-FODMAP lifestyle is not just about following a diet; it's about adopting a comprehensive approach to health that nourishes the body and soothes the gut. Thankfully, in today's digital age, you are not alone on this journey. The internet offers a wealth of resources to help guide you, from websites and blogs to apps, all designed to support your low-FODMAP journey.

When it comes to websites, there are numerous virtual portals that offer a wellspring of information about low-FODMAP living. For example, you can find dedicated health platforms that provide comprehensive overviews of the diet, scientific explanations of how it works, and updates on the latest research findings. These sites can be a great way to ground your knowledge in the solid bedrock of science.

Blogs, on the other hand, are where the low-FODMAP lifestyle truly comes to life. Personal accounts of individuals navigating the diet, coupled with creative, gut-friendly recipes, make blogs a valuable, relatable resource. Blogs often serve as a supportive community where experiences, advice, and encouragement are freely shared. You can find motivation and inspiration in the success stories of others, learn from their challenges, and discover ingenious ways to turn dietary restrictions into culinary opportunities.

As for apps, these are the handy companions for your low-FODMAP journey. Apps can offer personalized meal planning features, FODMAP food databases, and even grocery shopping assistants that help you decipher food labels. An app's portability also means you have a trove of low-FODMAP knowledge right in your pocket, making it easier to adhere to the diet, whether you're at the grocery store, at work, or dining out.

The beauty of these digital resources lies not just in the information they provide, but in the sense of community they foster. They underscore that you're not alone in your journey towards better gut health. Together, they provide a roadmap that can lead to a healthier, happier you – one low-FODMAP meal at a time.

Recommended Reading

Just as every individual is unique, so too is every journey through the world of low-FODMAP living. This journey is not simply about swapping one food for another but about education, understanding, and empowerment. Books, with their ability to dive deep into a subject, can be instrumental in this learning process. Here, we'll explore some recommended readings that could become your compass in navigating this diet.

If you're looking for a comprehensive guide that covers all the basics, consider "The Complete Low-FODMAP Diet" by Dr. Sue Shepherd and Dr. Peter Gibson. This book is often referred to as the 'Bible' of the low-FODMAP diet. Written by the very researchers who pioneered the diet, it offers detailed information about the science behind FODMAPs, along with practical advice, strategies, and recipes to guide you on your journey.

If recipes are your main interest, "The Low-FODMAP Recipe Book" by Lucy Whigham is a gem. This book can help you realize that adopting a low-FODMAP diet doesn't mean you're doomed to bland, boring meals. Instead, it can open a new culinary world filled with flavorful dishes that are both satisfying and gut-friendly.

For those interested in understanding the connection between gut health and overall wellbeing, "Gut: The Inside Story of Our Body's Most Underrated Organ" by Giulia Enders is a fascinating read. While it's not exclusively about the low-FODMAP diet, it offers valuable insights into the complex world inside our bellies and underscores the profound impact that our gut health can have on our lives.

If stress management is an area you'd like to explore alongside your diet, consider "The Stress Solution" by Dr. Rangan Chatterjee. It's well-established that stress can exacerbate IBS symptoms, and this book offers practical tools for achieving a more balanced, healthier lifestyle.

Finally, if you're seeking personal accounts and relatable experiences, Kate Scarlata's "The Low-FODMAP Diet Step by Step" provides a blend of scientific information, practical tips, and personal narratives. It beautifully captures the human side of the journey towards better gut health.

Remember, the journey towards a healthier you is a personal one, and different resources will resonate with different people. As you explore these recommended readings, find the voices that speak to you, and let them guide you in your pursuit of a more comfortable, healthier life. Just as a journey of a thousand miles begins with a single step, so too does your journey towards better gut health begin with a single page.

Chapter 13: Appendix: Low-FODMAP Food List

Detailed List of Low-FODMAP Foods

Starting a low-FODMAP diet can initially feel like navigating through a labyrinth, especially with the sheer amount of food options we're presented with in our daily lives. However, the world of low-FODMAP foods is far from limited or bland. It offers an array of delightful ingredients that can be used to create meals as varied, flavorful, and nourishing as any other diet.

When discussing low-FODMAP foods, it's essential to consider the different food groups, as each one has its unique options. Let's delve into these groups and unravel the diversity they offer.

Proteins: Proteins are the building blocks of our bodies and a crucial part of any diet. In the world of low-FODMAP, the options are numerous. Most meats and fish, including chicken, turkey, lamb, pork, beef, fish, and shellfish, are low in FODMAPs. Eggs are also a good source of protein and are FODMAP-friendly. For vegetarians and vegans, tofu and tempeh serve as excellent protein options.

Vegetables: Vegetables are often the most challenging category to handle when dealing with FODMAPs, as some of the most commonly consumed vegetables are high in FODMAPs. However, there are still plenty of choices. Bell peppers, carrots, cucumbers, eggplant, lettuce, olives, parsnips, potatoes, radishes, spinach, tomatoes, and zucchini are all good examples of low-FODMAP veggies.

Fruits: Fruits can be a minefield when it comes to FODMAPs, but several of them are on the friendly side. Bananas, blueberries, grapes, kiwi, oranges, pineapple, strawberries, and raspberries are all low in FODMAPs, allowing you to enjoy a naturally sweet treat without discomfort.

Dairy and Alternatives: Lactose, found in many dairy products, is a common FODMAP. Luckily, many dairy products come in lactose-free versions. Also, hard cheeses like cheddar and feta and aged cheeses like Parmesan are naturally low in lactose. For those who prefer plant-based options, almond milk, rice milk, and lactose-free soy milk are great alternatives.

Grains: Many people worry about missing out on grains when starting a low-FODMAP diet. However, several grains and cereals are low in FODMAPs, including quinoa, rice, oats, and corn. Some bread types, such as sourdough spelt bread and gluten-free bread, can also be included in a low-FODMAP diet.

Nuts and Seeds: While some nuts, like cashews and pistachios, are high in FODMAPs, many others can be enjoyed in moderation. Almonds, walnuts, macadamias, and peanuts are all low-FODMAP nuts. For seeds, pumpkin, sesame, and sunflower seeds are safe choices.

Remember, everyone's tolerance to FODMAPs is unique. It's not just about which foods to include, but also about portion sizes. Always listen to your body, as it's the best guide on this journey. The goal is not restriction but understanding your body's needs and preferences to create a diet that is healthy, enjoyable, and most importantly, comfortable for you. Let this be the start of your adventure into the flavorful and varied world of low-FODMAP foods.

Chapter 14: Index

Measurement conversion table

Measurement	Conversion
1 teaspoon (tsp)	5 milliliters (ml)
1 tablespoon (Tbsp)	15 milliliters (ml)
1 fluid ounce (fl oz)	30 milliliters (ml)
1 cup	240 milliliters (ml) / 8 fluid ounces (fl oz)
1 pint (pt)	2 cups / 480 milliliters (ml) / 16 fluid ounces (fl oz)
1 quart (qt)	2 pints (pt) / 32 fluid ounces (fl oz) / 0.946 liters (l)
1 gallon (gal)	4 quarts (qt) / 128 fluid ounces (fl oz) / 3.785 liters (l)
1 ounce (oz)	28.35 grams (g)
1 pound (lb)	16 ounces (oz) / 454 grams (g)
1 kilogram (kg)	2.204 pounds (lb) / 35.27 ounces (oz)

Temperature conversion table

Fahrenheit (°F)	Celsius (°C)
32°F	0°C
50°F	10°C
68°F	20°C
86°F	30°C
104°F	40°C
122°F	50°C
140°F	60°C
158°F	70°C
176°F	80°C
194°F	90°C
212°F	100°C

www.ingramcontent.com/pod-product-compliance
Lightning Source LLC
Chambersburg PA
CBHW080812280726
48660CB00018B/3279